Pictures Worth a 100 Points™

2nd Edition

A Concise Pictorial Review
for the Pediatric Board Review

By Stu Silverstein, MD

Illustrations by Jaime Phalen, MD, FAAP

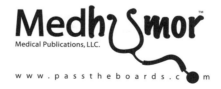

MedHumor
Medical Publications, LLC.

www.passtheboards.com

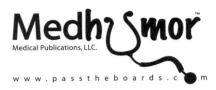

Medhumor Medical Publications, LLC
Stamford, Connecticut

Printed in the United States of America

*This book is designed to provide information and guidance in regard to the subject matter covered.
It is to be used as a study guide for physicians preparing for the United States Medical Licensing Examination (USMLE™) which is sponsored by the Federation of State Medical Boards (FSMB) of the United States, Inc., and the National Board of Medical Examiners ® (NBME®). It is not meant to be a clinical manual. The reader is advised to consult textbooks and other reference manuals in making clinical decisions. It is not the purpose of this book to reprint all the information that is otherwise available, but rather to assist the Board Candidate in organizing the material to facilitate study and recall on the exam. The reader is encouraged to read other sources of material, in particular picture atlases that are available.*

Although every precaution has been taken in the preparation of this book, the publisher, author, and members of the editorial board assume no responsibility for errors, omissions or typographical mistakes.   Neither is any liability assumed for damages resulting from the direct and indirect use of the information contained herein. The book contains information that is up-to-date only up to the printing date. Due to the very nature of the medical profession, there will be points out-of-date as soon as the book rolls off the press. The purpose of this book is to educate and entertain.

**If you do not wish to be bound by the above,
you may return this book to the publisher for a full refund.**

Publisher: MedHumor Medical Publications, LLC
                        Stamford, CT.

Senior Editor: Stu Silverstein, MD
                        Author, *"Laughing Your Way to Passing the Pediatric Boards"*
                        www.passtheboards.com

Medical Illustrations: Jaime Phalen, MD, FAAP

Design / Copy Editor: Antoinette D'Amore, A.D. Design
                             www.addesign-graphics.com

Cover Designer: Rachel Mindrup
                        www.rmindrup.com

About the Author

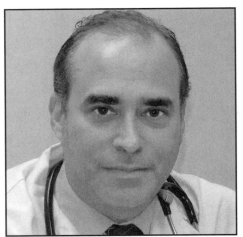

Dr. Stu Silverstein is the founder and CEO of Medhumor Medical Publications, LLC which began with the publication of the critically acclaimed "Laughing your way to Passing the Pediatric Boards"™ back in the spring of 2000. Word spread quickly that finally there was a book out there that turned a traditionally daunting process into one that was actually fun and enjoyable. This groundbreaking study guide truly "took the boredom out of board review"® with reports from our readers that they were able to spend half the time studying while retaining twice the material.

The concept of the "Laughing your way to Passing the Boards"™ and Medhumor Medical Publications, LLC were conceived by Dr. Silverstein. He brought his years of experience in the field of Standup Comedy and Comedy writing after he realized the critical need for a study guide that spoke the language of colleagues rather than the language of dusty textbooks. His work as a Standup Comedian and Medical Humorist has frequently been featured in several newspapers, radio programs and TV shows, including the New York Times, WCBC newsradio in NY City, as well as World News Tonight with Peter Jennings.

Dr. Silverstein is also a contributing editor for the <u>Resident and Staff Physician</u> annual board review issue and has authored numerous articles on medical humor. He has served on the faculty of the Osler Institute Board Review course and for the UCLA Pediatric Board Review course. He is the co-author of "What about Me? Growing up with a Developmentally Disabled Sibling" written with Dr. Bryna Siegel, professor of Child Psychiatry , UCSF.

Dr. Silverstein is a popular lecturer at residency programs, once again helping residents "take the boredom out of their board review"®.

Dr. Silverstein is the Clinical Director of Firefly After Hours Pediatrics, LLC, an after hours pediatrics specializing in after hours acute care pediatrics. Dr. Silverstein is also an attending physician with Our Lady or Mercy Medical Center in the Bronx and is a Clinical Assistant Professor of Emergency Medicine at the New York Medical College in Valhalla, NY.

The 2nd Edition

You will notice some dramatic changes in our 2nd edition of "Pictures worth 100 Points".

In response to reader feedback we have added an entire section devoted to color drawings.

In addition we have eliminated the quiz section.

So many of you have written to us regarding how helpful the 1st edition was in passing the general pediatric board exam. We hope that by adding additional drawings and entire section this 2nd edition will be even more helpful.

As always we appreciate any and all feedback from those who have used our materials.

Sincerely,

Stuart C. Silverstein, MD
Stamford , Connecticut

This book is once again dedicated to my children, Isra and Daniel and the newest addition baby boy Ariel, whose very existence gives life meaning and keeps things in perspective. Every day they remind me that it is never too late to have a happy childhood.

Acknowledgments

I would like to thank my wife Dr. Guita Sazan for standing behind me at all times. Her strength and love is the nourishment that feeds my life.

I would also like to acknowledge my children: Isra, Daniel and Ariel. They have all taught me that it is never too late to have a 2nd childhood.

I would like to acknowledge my parents, Beverly and Richard Silverstein, for their inspiration early in my life by teaching me the importance of education and discipline.

Without the help of our General Manager Todd Van Allen this project would never stay on track and you would be holding a ream of paper in your hand rather than a book.

Dr. Jaime Phalen's unique talent and work ethic has been invaluable as we look forward to working with and learning from him in the future.

Antoinette D'Amore's unique skills in layout and design were instrumental in the look of this and all of our books and publications

Stuart C. Silverstein, MD
Medhumor Medical Publications, LLC
Stamford, CT

Table of Contents

Signposts for Pictures Worth a 100 Points™

You will notice throughout the text signposts in the left margin. These signposts are there to help navigate the material in a more organized and focused fashion.

They will also help when you go back to review specific material that you wish to focus on.

These signposts indicate the following

Definition –This points to a specific definition of a term. This is important since definitions are very specific and by knowing these specifics you are less likely to be tricked on the exam.
For example Ventricular Tachycardia is defined as 150-240 beats per minute in adults.

Insider Tips – This points to a particular bit of information that is crucial to passing the exam.

Peril – Watch out for this slippery when wet sign. Those who ignore it do so at their own peril since this points to important *tricks that previous exam takers have fallen for*.

Buzz Words – These phrases are important to note since there are only a limited number of ways a disorder or disease can be described. Often the wording will be the same and this sign post calls attention to such phrases.

Look For – Similar to the phrase that pays this indicates specific findings and signs you should look at in a picture or imaging study that often "gives the answer away".

Mnemonic – Easy ways to remember important facts are located next to this icon.

Either Or Choices – Many times on the exam you will be down to two choices.
Frequently 1-2 important facts distinguish one clinical condition from another. Follow this signpost for specific examples where one factor distinguished the correct choice from the wrong choice.

Picture Perfect:
Preparing for the Photo and Graphic Section of the Exam

Photo Sensitive

Beginning with the 2008 exam the pictures will no longer be limited to one booklet on day 2 of the exam.

In fact the exam has now been compressed into one day which will allow you to de-compress a lot sooner.

However the approach to the photos and graphics should remain the same.

The Curve Ball

They pretty much know how imaging studies are presented in typical pediatric textbooks you are using to prepare for the exam. Therefore, they will often present a "different look" or a "different angle" than is usually used in popular picture books.

For example, the typical photo seen in many texts of "trichotillomania" is long hair with streaks of missing hair in the back. One year they showed a child with short hair.

Change the Angle

I recall one x-ray that I could not for the life of me figure out. I literally crossed my eyes, the way I did in Kindergarten to escape the boredom, to see if the image would appear. I finally turned the image on its side, and sure enough, the image was obvious.

Look at the pictures from a variety of angles to see what they are getting at. There is nothing there by accident. If they show you tape around the upper lip, they are telling you "the child was extubated."

Hey Look up Here, Not Down There!

On occasion you will be focusing on the wrong part of the picture and miss the diagnostic tree while viewing the forest. Sometimes just the opposite will happen.

I recall a neonatal x-ray on the exam. I crossed my eyes, crossed my toes, and finally crossed my teeth, but the abdominal and chest both looked normal. Finally I noticed the fractured clavicle and THAT was the key to the answer. By focusing on the abdominal –pulmonary forest I almost missed the clavicular tree. Another question featured a child who had what I thought was a vague rash, nothing much more than that. I looked up and down and noticed that the child looked "Japanese" and wallah, it hit me: "Kawasaki Disease", and then the conjunctivitis and other signs became obvious.

Easy with Asymmetry

Don't forget to look for asymmetry. Often, this is the key to the answer. For example, they could show a picture and *asymmetry* is all you see. Then the word *"hemihypertrophy"* will pop out at you.

Don't forget to write a description of the physical findings in the margins when you spot them. Chances are you studied the descriptive words, so writing the description words jogs your memory and increases the chances of you tapping into your study time.

Prepping for Pictures: Preparing for the Picture Section

"Conventional Wisdom" for Board preparation states: "Just look over some pictures a week or 2 before the exam and you'll recognize it when you see it." **WRONG!** You need to have a systematic approach to studying the picture section.

Differentiating the Differences

Some examples you will need to distinguish are:

❑ Glaucoma vs. Cataracts
❑ Trichotillomania vs. Alopecia
❑ Areata vs. Tinea Capitis

The Devil is to Know the Differences on Which to Really Focus

Like most of the test, the key is in the minor differences between similar disorders. Prepare a list of disorders that appear similar but have slight differences.

Not Just Looking

Just "looking over the photos" won't cut it. You need a system to study the photos and graphic depictions. Here are some suggestions:

Integrate and Coordinate

- Integrate picture studying with each section. Note differences between similar disorders and syndromes and what makes them different.

Captain's Log

- Maintain a log of what you are to specifically look for in each picture. Do this in a notebook.

Photo Days

- Set aside 2 – 3 weeks toward the end specifically for photos and other graphics. In doing so, you will automatically be reviewing all previously studied sections.

Getting Down to Specifics

The chapters in this book are broken down by type of imaging study and part of the body since this is how you will encounter themo on the exam. This will allow you to methodically consider what they are showing you on the exam when you see a photo or an imaging study.

Here is where knowing the specific differences that separate one disorder from another really helps.

While studying the images in this book you should look at the pictures focusing on the specific features on which you will be tested.

Section 1:
Picture Perfect
Black & White

Dermatology

Psoriasis

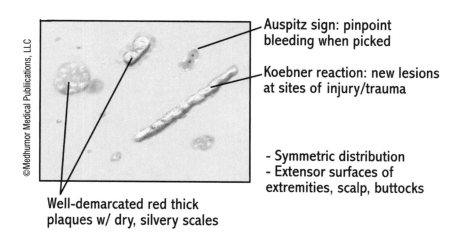

Auspitz sign: pinpoint bleeding when picked

Koebner reaction: new lesions at sites of injury/trauma

- Symmetric distribution
- Extensor surfaces of extremities, scalp, buttocks

©Medhumor Medical Publications, LLC

Well-demarcated red thick plaques w/ dry, silvery scales

- Chronic, relapsing, inflammatory disease
- Strong genetic basis
- Risk factors: Eastern European or Scandinavian, female, 16-22 y/o

Psoriasis has a symmetric distribution, on the extensor surfaces of extremities. It can be found on the scalp and buttocks as well.

Look for well demarcated, red, thick plaques with dry silvery scales

Auspitz Sign is an important subtle illustration they might present. It is what is left behind when the silvery plaque associated with psoriasis is picked off.

A history of relapses is typical and they might describe it in other family members.

The rash often appears at sites of trauma which is known as **Koebner phenomenon**. *Pitted nails* are also often part of the description.

Guttate psoriasis is a variant of psoriasis. It consists of small drop like scaly plaques on the trunk and extremities, usually following a strep infection.

Capillary (Strawberry) Hemangioma

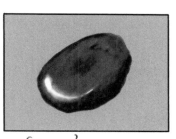
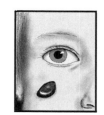

- Polyploid raised, bright red to deep purple lesions
- Present at or shortly after birth
- Most common on head

These are polypoid raised lesions usually bright red to deep purple in color.

They are typically seen shortly after birth most commonly on the head or face

Strawberry hemangiomas are also called *capillary hemangiomas* go through a rapid growth period before they involute. Don't be fooled into believing this is a malignancy if this is emphasized in the history. In other words capillary hemangiomas get worse before they get better.

Cavernous hemangiomas can be confused with strawberry hemangiomas. However, with cavernous hemangiomas the vessels are larger, located deeper and are bluer than the red strawberry hemangioma.

Treatment is reserved for cases that:

- Interfere with vision
- Involve the spinal cord or brain
- Interfere with the airway

Kasabach-Merritt syndrome occurs when there is a rapidly enlarging deep hemangioma resulting in trapping of platelets and coagulation factors.

This can lead to a coagulopathy secondary to DIC as well as thrombocytopenia and hemolytic anemia.

Pitryriasis Rosea

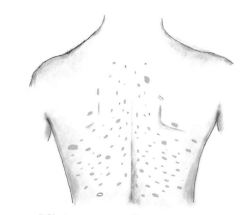

©Medhumor Medical Publications, LLC

Tinea versicolor
↓
hypopigmentel
Shreaded patch
M. furfur
Se sulfich

"Christmas tree" pattern on back

- Oval lesions oriented along dermal lines
- Lesions may be macular, raised, or scaly

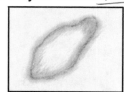

- "Herald patch"
  --Signals onset, appearing on trunk/thigh
  --Large, isolated, salmon-colored, scaly
  --Often mistaken for tinea corporis

Look for the classic **Christmas tree pattern** *on the back.* **Oval lesions** oriented along dermal likes of the back.

Look for

The lesions may be described as or shown to be:
- Macular
- Raises
- Scaly

The classic finding is the **herald patch** which is seen in the beginning of the rash, and "heralds" its onset. The herald patch is typically seen on the trunk or thigh.

It is large salmon colored and scaly

Think of it as an actual salmon, its association with the Christmas tree distribution and its being a herald patch. Now picture a giant Christmas tree on Herald Square with scaly, smelly salmon ornaments on the trunk.

Dermoid Cyst

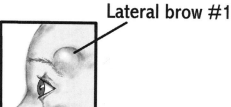

Lateral brow #1

Smooth, mobile, nontender, subcutaneous mass

DEFINITION

Smooth, mobile, non tender, subcutaneous mass

Location , Mobility and Sensitivity

Characteristics - smooth

Mobility – mobile

Tender – non tender

Location – subcutaneous on face but can be seen elsewhere and if in the midline or the spine beware

Treatment is surgical excision.

PERIL

WARNING

If midline especially spinal, an MRI must be ordered to rule out communication with the spinal tract.

Normal Scalp

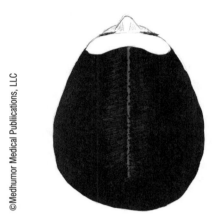

Normal Scalp with full head of hair before preparing for and taking the board exam

Alopecia Areata

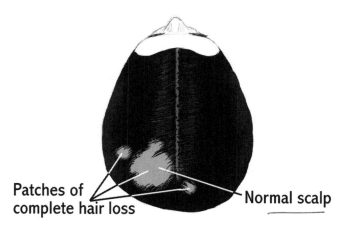

©Medhumor Medical Publications, LLC

Patches of
complete hair loss

Normal scalp

Short, easily-pulled
hairs at margins

The hair loss of alopecia is most likely due to an autoimmune disorder

Patches of complete hair loss without erythema, scaling skin or broken hairs. The onset is sudden and often the hair that comes in lacks pigment.

Short easily pulled hairs at the margins is one of the hallmarks of alopecia areata

Tinea capitis is characterized by erythema , scaling skin and broken hairs. As noted above these characteristics are not seen in alopecia areata **Traction alopecia** can be distinguished since the bald patches are limited to areas of physical stress, i.e. braided hair.

Alopecia totalis as the name implies is total hair loss including eyebrows and eyelashes.

It does *not* include the loss of pubic hair and chest hair but let's face this is something unlikely to appear on the exam Let's hope not!

Universalis

Trichotillomania

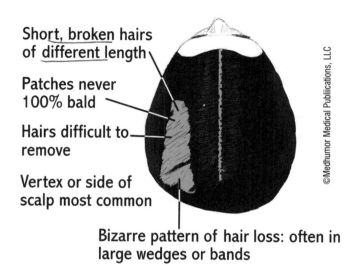

Short, broken hairs of <u>different length</u>

Patches never 100% bald

Hairs difficult to remove

Vertex or side of scalp most common

Bizarre pattern of hair loss: often in large wedges or bands

©Medhumor Medical Publications, LLC

Short broken hairs of different length. The most common spot to be involved is the vertex or side of the scalp. Look for bizarre patterns of hair loss, often in large wedges or bands

Patches are <u>never</u> 100% bald

Think of the vertex as the easiest place to grab hair.

Tinea Capitis

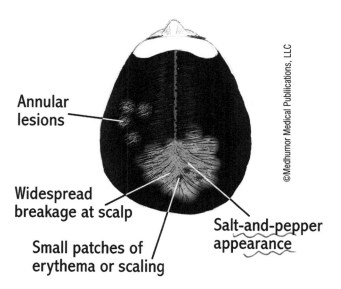

Annular lesions

Widespread breakage at scalp

Small patches of erythema or scaling

Salt-and-pepper appearance

©Medhumor Medical Publiications, LLC

- Annular lesions
- Widespread breakage at the scalp
- Salt and Pepper appearance
- Small patches of erythema or scaling

Alopecia Totalis

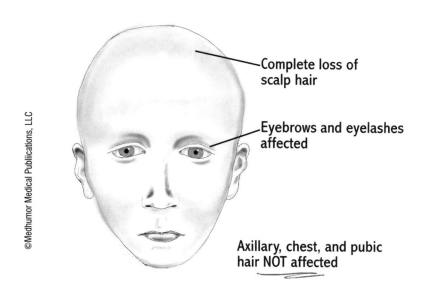

Complete loss of scalp hair

Eyebrows and eyelashes affected

Axillary, chest, and pubic hair NOT affected

©Medhumor Medical Publications, LLC

Alopecia totalis as the name implies is total hair loss including eyebrows and eyelashes.

 It does not include the loss of pubic hair and chest hair.

Acanthosis Nigricans

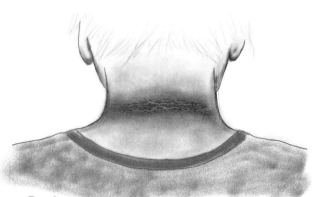

- Dark, velvety thickened skin lesion in flexures: posterior neck, axillae, and groin
- #1 cause: obesity +/- insulin resistance
- More common in dark-skinned races

Acanthosis nigricans is associated with insulin resistance and thus type 2 diabetes. It is more common in dark pigmented skin.

The drawing depicts dark velvety skin in the folds of the neck. It can also appear in axilla and groin.

Hypomelanotic Macule

"Ash-leaf spot"

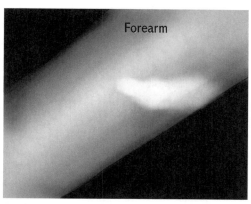

- Typically the earliest skin manifestation
- More than three = specific (DIAGNOSTIC)

The drawing depicts classic hypomelanotic macules or " ash leaf spots" as they are commonly known in major texts.

- Hypomelanotic macules (ash leaf spots) are the earliest manifestation of tuberous sclerosis.
- The spots are more prominent when viewed in ultraviolet light (Woods lamp).
- The presence of more than three is a major diagnostic criterion for tuberous sclerosis.

Shagreen Patch

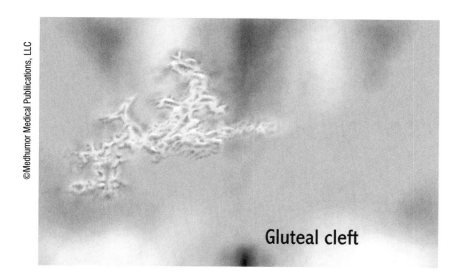

Gluteal cleft

The drawing depicts the shagreen patch associated with tuberous sclerosis

The features include the following:

- Firm yellowish-red or pink area of nodules
- Orange peel or cobblestone texture
- In patients with tuberous sclerosis the shagreen patch is nearly always found on or around the lumbar region of back

ENT

Cholesteatoma

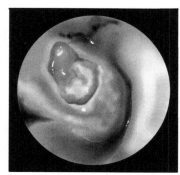

©Medhumor Medical Publications, LLC

- Trapped squamous epithelium
- Growth beneath TM
- Causes: congenital, TM retraction, trauma
- #1 symptom: painless otorrhea
- #1 sign: perf'd TM w/ drainage and granulation tissue
- Sequelae: Bony erosion, hearing loss
- If in doubt, get CT scan

Cholesteatoma is the result of the accumulation of keratinized squamous epithelium.

Cholesteatoma presents as *painless otorrhea, drainage of white , shiny debris and granulation tissue* resulting in boney erosion and hearing loss. Malodorous discharge will also be described in the history.

Cholesteatoma is diagnosed by CT scan

Cystic Hygroma
aka Lymphangioma

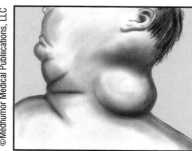

Soft sac-like neck mass with indistinct borders

Benign, multiloculated, cystic structure filled w/ lymph

Frequently involves neurovascular structures

Neck #1 site

2/3 noted at birth

Complications:
- Airway obstruction
- Bleeding
- Infection

Hint: Chromosomal anomalies
- Turner syndrome (46,XO) #1
- Trisomy 13, 18, or 21

Cystic Hygroma is a lymphangioma or a benign, multiloculated cystic structure filled with lymph. You should recognize one when you see one even across a large filled to capacity auditorium.

Massive swelling on the side of the neck *without discoloration*. The borders are indistinct.

Complications include:

- *Airway obstruction*
- *Bleeding*
- *Infection*

Cystic hygroma is associated with Turner Syndrome and Trisomy 13

Auricular Hematoma

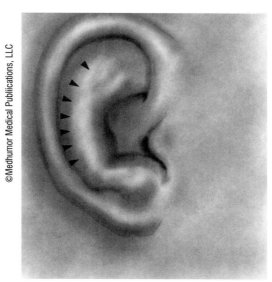

©Medhumor Medical Publications, LLC

Emergency I&D

In addition to being expected to recognize the auricular hematoma you will be expected to know that prompt surgical evacuation of the hematoma is required to avoid a cauliflower deformity.

An auricular hematoma is usually due to blunt trauma to the ear, often occurring in teenagers who are wrestling.

Genetics

Hallermann-Streiff Syndrome

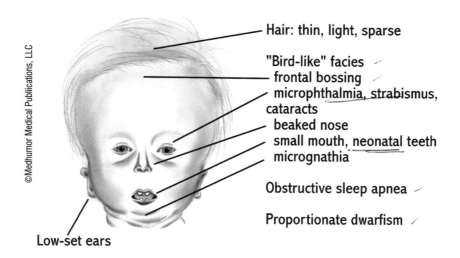

©Medhumor Medical Publications, LLC

Hair: thin, light, sparse

"Bird-like" facies
frontal bossing
microphthalmia, strabismus,
cataracts
beaked nose
small mouth, neonatal teeth
micrognathia

Obstructive sleep apnea

Proportionate dwarfism

Low-set ears

Hint: look for eyeglasses and bird-like face

Pointed nose, bird like face including small eyes.

They will typically show a child wearing glasses and a bird like face.

They also look a bit like hockey star, Wayne Gretzky, which should help one remember the neonatal teeth.

Ectodermal Dysplasia

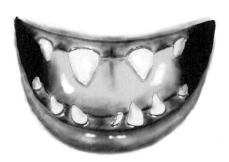

- Peg-shaped, pointed, or missing teeth
- Defective enamel
- Dentures as early as two years of age

A smile only a mother[1] could love…

Children with both ectodermal dysplasia and Hallermann Streiff can present with defective teeth, watch for the description or picture of the difference

Children with **ectodermal hypoplasia** has:

- Peg teeth
- Pointed teeth / missing teeth
- Hypoplastic nails
- Fine sparse hair
- Abnormalities of sweat and sebaceous glands

Dentures is another common feature

Children with **Hallermann Streiff** have neonatal teeth

---

[1] Or Grandpa from the Munsters

Hemihypertrophy + Aniridia

©Medhumor Medical Publications, LLC

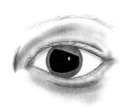

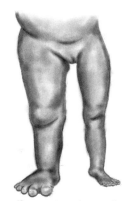

Aniridia = hereditary, congenital, severe iris hypoplasia

Hemihypertrophy = Asymmetric overgrowth of the skull, face, trunk, or extremities, +/- visceral involvement.

Associated syndromes:
- WAGR: Wilms tumor, Aniridia, Genitourinary anomalies, mental Retardation
- Beckwith-Wiedeman
- Silver-Russel
- Proteus: This is what Joseph Merrick (The Elephant Man) had!

Hemihypertrophy and aniridia are associated with the following syndromes:
- WAGR[2]
- Wilms Tumor
- Beckwith – Wiedemann Syndrome
- Silver Russell Syndrome

Hemihypertrophy and aniridia are associated with the following findings:
- Genitourinary Anomalies
- Mental Retardation

Hemihypertrophy is what Joseph Merrick, more commonly know as the Elephant Man, had.

---

[2] WAGR = Wilms tumor, Aniridia, Genitourinary anomalies, and mental Retardation

They will describe a child with one half of the body being larger than the other or showing it. They will rarely if ever use the word hemihypertrophy.

Lesch-Nyhan Syndrome
X-linked recessive

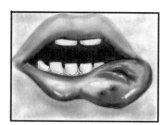

Self-injurious behavior:
- Biting -> partial amputation of digits, tongue, lips
- Hitting/abrasion -> scarring, injury
- Compulsive spitting, hitting, cursing

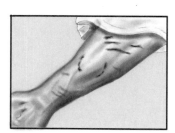

©Medhumor Medical Publications, LLC

Key clinical elements:
- overproduction of uric acid
- neurological disability
- behavioral problems

LOOK FOR Since self mutilation is an important component they will typically present a child with *partially amputated digits, tongue and lips.*

LOOK FOR If they present you with a child with a history of compulsive hitting, spitting and cursing, they are either describing a child with Lesch Nyhan Syndrome or the 3rd quarter of an NBA basketball game.

EITHER OR CHOICES Cursing and "coprolalia" can be a part of Tourette syndrome however the other components of Lesch Nyhan will not be presented if the correct diagnosis is Tourette Syndrome.

Elevated uric acid levels are an important part of the history to note and therefore Gout can be part of the presentation of a patient with Lesch-Nyhan Syndrome.

In addition, *choreiform movements* can be a part of the presenting history.

Orange-colored crystal-like deposits (orange sand) in the child's diaper can be the first symptom to appear.

Werdnig-Hoffman Syndrome
aka Infantile Spinal Muscular Atrophy (SMA) Type 1

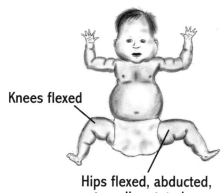

Knees flexed

Hips flexed, abducted, externally rotated

- Onset in first 6 months

- Progressive, symmetrical muscle weakness

- Proximal worse than distal

- Severe hypotonia w/ absent DTRs

- Death by 2 yrs, usually from respiratory failure

Hint: Look for "floppy baby" w/ suck, swallow, breathing problems (tracheostomy)

Hint: Tongue fasciculations are pathognomonic!

They will typically present an infant younger than 6months with symmetrical muscle weakness starting with proximal muscles. *Deep tendon reflexes will be absent*

If they describe *tongue fasciculations* look no further - you have your diagnosis.

Watch for an infant with a tracheostomy.

The poor suck/swallow will also be described in **infantile botulism toxicity**. If the diagnosis is Werdnig-Hoffman syndrome they will be obligated to describe the other associated findings.

With botulism toxicity; the infant the *poor suck/swallow will be of sudden onset*, not gradual.

Cornelia de Lange Syndrome

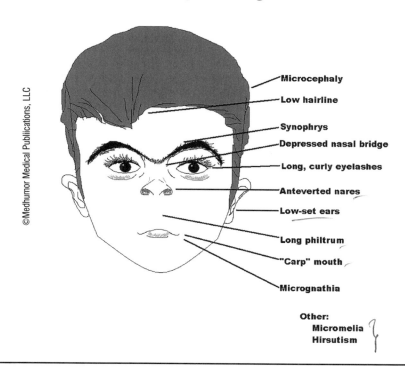

©Medhumor Medical Publications, LLC

- Microcephaly
- Low hairline
- Synophrys
- Depressed nasal bridge
- Long, curly eyelashes
- Anteverted nares
- Low-set ears
- Long philtrum
- "Carp" mouth
- Micrognathia

Other:
Micromelia
Hirsutism

Hair is the main theme with this and if you remember this point you will recognize this syndrome which will certainly appear in the picture section of the exam

Hair features include:

- Low hairline
- Long curly eyelashes
- Hirsutism
- Synophrys[4]

Note! - A non specific finding seen in other disorders would be low set ears.[3]

Other features include the **3 micros**:

- Micro*cephaly*
- Micro*gnathia*
- Micro*melia* [5]

---

[3] When dealing with a very common feature, you may wish to ignore it when reading the question and focus on the more specific findings being presented.

[4] Eyebrows that meet in the middle

[5] Abnormal smallness of the limbs

Look for other **mouth features**:
- Carp Mouth
- Long Philtrum
- Anteverted nares

Pierre-Robin Syndrome

©Medhumor Medical Publications, LLC

CNS defects (50%)

Auricular anomalies (75%)

Otitis media 80%

CLASSIC TRIAD:
Cleft palate (14-91%)
Glossoptosis (70-85%)
Micrognathia (92%)

Musculoskeletal
anomalies (70-80%)

The classic triad of **Pierre –Robin Syndrome** are:

1. Cleft Palate
2. Glossoptosis
3. Micrognathia

Additional features include:

- CNS abnormalities
- Ear Abnormalities
- Musculoskeletal abnormalities
- Palate – cleft or arched

Maintenance of airway can be difficult if the child is not prone

Noonan Syndrome

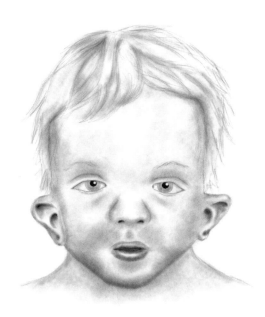

©Medhumor Medical Publications, LLC

M:F

 The facial features of Noonan syndrome depicted in the drawing include:

- Webbed neck (short broad neck with skin folds)
- Drooping eyelids
- Downward slanting of the eyes
- Arched eyebrows
- Redundant skin fold / inner angle of the eyes
- Wide spaced eyes
- Flat broad root of the nose
- Low set ears
- Triangular face

Additional features include

- Aortic stenosis
- Undescended testicles

To differentiate cardiac lesions of Noonan (left sided lesion) from Turner (right sided lesion) syndromes, you might consider the following mnemonic.

---

6 Or Face for those who prefer English over Latin

Turner Syndrome

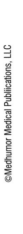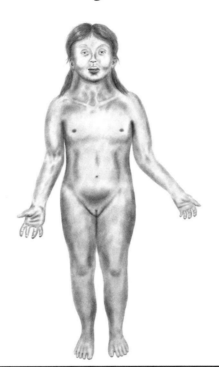

©Medhumor Medical Publications, LLC

female hypogonadism

The illustration demonstrates some of the features of Turner Syndrome including:

- Short stature
- Low hairline
- Wide spaced nipples
- Shortened metacarpal
- Shield shaped chest
- Brown nevi
- Fold of skin on neck
- Elbow deformity
- Underdeveloped gonads

Short

Trisomy 13 and 18

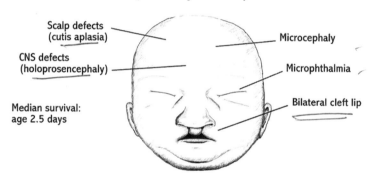

Trisomy 18
(Edward syndrome)

Characteristic hand posture

Index finger
overlaps middle

5th finger
overlaps 4th

Hypoplastic
nails

Clenched hand

Trisomy 13 and 18

Rocker-Bottom Foot

Prominent calcaneus

Trisomy 13
(Patau syndrome)

Scalp defects
(cutis aplasia)

CNS defects
(holoprosencephaly)

Median survival:
age 2.5 days

Microcephaly

Microphthalmia

Bilateral cleft lip

Trisomy 18

DEFINITION

Trisomy 18 is also known as Edward syndrome

LOOK FOR

Look for *rocker bottom feet, horseshoe kidneys, clenched fist with overlapping fingers* in addition to the common features below.

Trisomy 13

Trisomy 13 is also known as Patau syndrome

Look for *cleft lip/palate, polydactyly,* and *holoprosencephaly* in addition to the common features below.

An important feature includes scalp defects especially in the occipto-parietal area. This may be the only feature they might show you.

Both in Common

Mental retardation and congenital heart disease

Sturge-Weber Syndrome

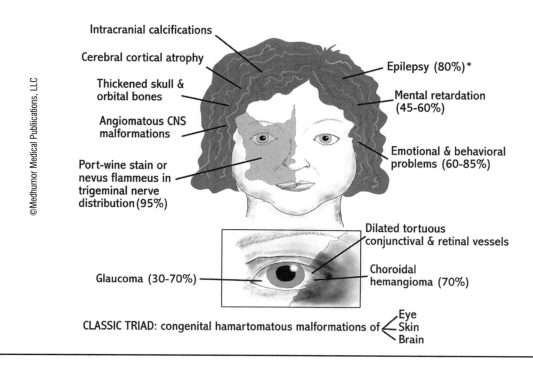

Intracranial calcifications

Cerebral cortical atrophy

Thickened skull & orbital bones

Angiomatous CNS malformations

Port-wine stain or nevus flammeus in trigeminal nerve distribution (95%)

Epilepsy (80%)*

Mental retardation (45-60%)

Emotional & behavioral problems (60-85%)

Dilated tortuous conjunctival & retinal vessels

Glaucoma (30-70%)

Choroidal hemangioma (70%)

©Medhumor Medical Publications, LLC

CLASSIC TRIAD: congenital hamartomatous malformations of ← Eye, Skin, Brain

The classic triad of Sturge Weber Sydnrome consists of eye, brain and skin manifestations as outlined in the table below.

Location	Physical Exam	Imaging Study	History
Head	Facial Port Wine Stain	Intracranial Calcifications Cortical Atrophy	Seizures Mental Retardation Behavioral problems
Eyes	Torturous retinal vessels Glaucoma Choroidal hemangioma	—	—

The inheritance pattern of Sturge Weber Syndrome is random.

The port wine stain typically involves distribution of the 1st and 2nd branches of trigeminal nerves. For those of you who may have forgotten microdetails of gross anatomy you can continue to watch Gross Anatomy rather than dusting off your old copy of the show's namesake.

They will need to demonstrate the port wine stain covering at least one upper eyelid and the surrounding forehead.

When Sturge Weber is suspected a screening MRI is mandatory. Patients need to be followed by ophthalmology to measure intraocular pressure due to the risk for glaucoma.

Hutchinson-Gilford Progeria Syndrome (Progeria)

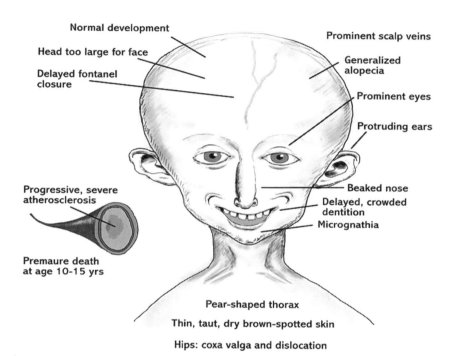

©Medhumor Medical Publications, LLC

Normal development

Head too large for face

Delayed fontanel closure

Prominent scalp veins

Generalized alopecia

Prominent eyes

Protruding ears

Progressive, severe atherosclerosis

Premaure death at age 10-15 yrs

Beaked nose

Delayed, crowded dentition

Micrognathia

Pear-shaped thorax

Thin, taut, dry brown-spotted skin

Hips: coxa valga and dislocation

Incidence: very rare
Inheritance: autosomal dominant

The essential feature is premature aging.

When looking at the key features, consider the features of an old person and it is easy to remember them.

From head to toe, look for the following features

Head –

- Generalized alopecia with a head too large for face
- Protruding ears and prominent eyes
- Prominent scalp veins
- Small lower Face Small chin, crowded teeth and small beak like nose

Thorax –

- Thin chest with brown spots

Hips –

- Dislocated hips frequently a problem

 Think of Mr. Smithers Homer's boss on the hit show The Simpsons®

 They have premature atherosclerosis resulting in premature death in the 2nd decade of life.

Waardenburg Syndrome

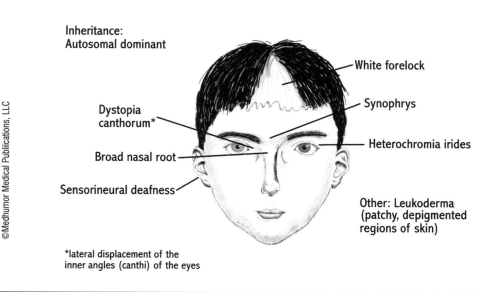

Inheritance:
Autosomal dominant

White forelock

©Medhumor Medical Publications, LLC

Dystopia
canthorum*

Synophrys

Broad nasal root

Heterochromia irides

Sensorineural deafness

Other: Leukoderma
(patchy, depigmented
regions of skin)

*lateral displacement of the
inner angles (canthi) of the eyes

The key features to remember in order to recognize this on the exam are
   1) White Forelock
   2) Heterochromic iris[1]
   3) Sensorineural deafness

Remember it is sensorineural deafness not obstructive.

If these findings weren't enough look for lateral displacement of the inner canthi of the eye.

The white forelock[2] is actually part of *partial albinism* seen in the syndrome therefore you can also look for :
   • Hypopigmented fundi noted
   • Depigmented areas of skin[3]

Waardenburg is inherited in an *autosomal dominant* pattern

---

[1] In somebody not using those over the counter combination contact lens, key ring, can opener jobs available at cashier checkout lines.
[2] A medical pompous way of saying white hair in the front.
[3] Hmm, different colored eyes, white patches, perhaps the Michael Jackson puzzle is coming together,? ... Nah!

Menkes Kinky Hair Syndrome
X-linked disorder of copper metabolism

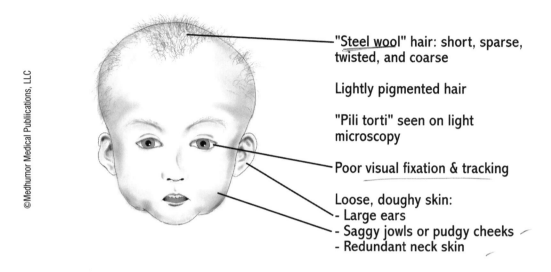

©Medhumor Medical Publications, LLC

"Steel wool" hair: short, sparse, twisted, and coarse

Lightly pigmented hair

"Pili torti" seen on light microscopy

Poor visual fixation & tracking

Loose, doughy skin:
- Large ears
- Saggy jowls or pudgy cheeks
- Redundant neck skin

Progressive neurodegeneration -> death by age 3 yrs

DEFINITION

Menkes Kinky Hair Syndrome is an X- Linked disorder of Copper Metabolism resulting in a decreased serum cooper/ceruloplasmin level

LOOK FOR

If presented with a picture of a child with Menkes Kinky Hair Syndrome, the photo must include the following features which will be apparent

- " Steel Wool Hair " which consists of short , sparse twisted , and coarse hair
- Doughy Skin
- Large Ears
- Saggy Jowels or Pudgy cheeks
- Redundant neck Skin
- Lightly Pigmented hair
- Pili Torti seen under microscope[1]

---

[1] This is just another way or perhaps once again it is Latin for twisted hair seen on microscopic exam

The history will include poor visual fixation and tracking. Death is typical by age 3 so if they present a patient older than 3 this is probably not the diagnosis.

Seizures, hypotonia, hypothermia and mental retardation can also be a part of the presenting history.

Sounds a lot like Larry from the 3 Stooges.

Reiter Syndrome

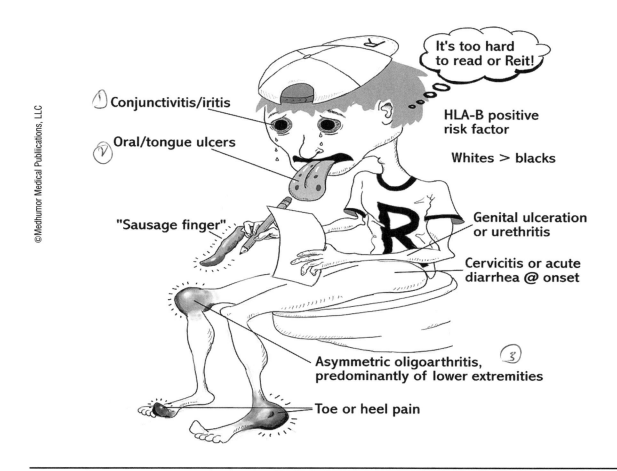

Can be remembered with the classic mnemonic
    Can't pee
    Can't See
    And it hurts in my knee

Beckwith-Wiedemann Syndrome

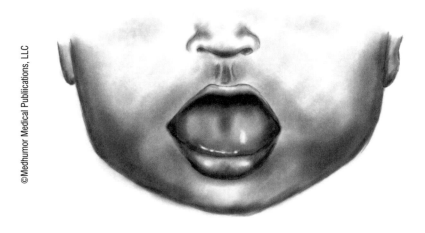

©Medhumor Medical Publications, LLC

Cardinal features: EMG triad
- Exomphalos
- Macroglossia
- Gigantism

Charge Syndrome

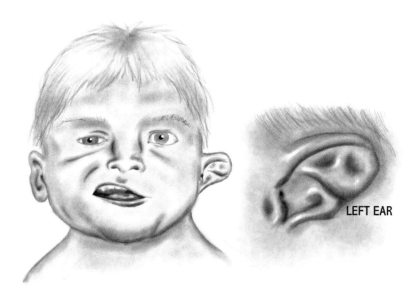

©Medhumor Medical Publications, LLC

LEFT EAR

CHARGE is of course stands for

- Coloboma of the eye
- Heart defect
- Atresia of the choanae
- Retardation of growth and/or development
- Genital hypoplasia
- Ear malformations

It is the additional facial features which are depicted in this drawing including:

- Facial paralysis or palsy
- Square shape of the face and head
- Flat cheekbones (malar hypoplasia)
- Facial asymmetry
- Wide nose with a high bridge
- Characteristic malformed protruding ear (ipsilateral to facial palsy)

In the ear drawing please note that :

- The "CHARGE ear" is short and wide ear with little or no lobe

Fetal Alcohol Syndrome

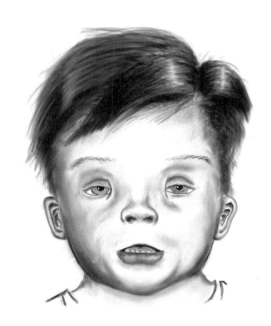

©Medhumor Medical Publications, LLC

DIAGNOSTIC facial features:
- Shortened palpebral fissures
- Smooth philtrum
- Thin upper lip

Associated facial features:
- Ptosis
- Epicanthal folds
- Short, upturned nose
- "Railroad track" ears
- Midfacial hypoplasia
- Micrognathia

Fetal Hydantoin Syndrome

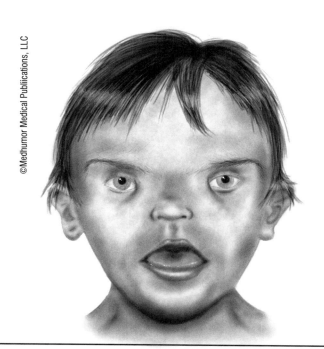

©Medhumor Medical Publications, LLC

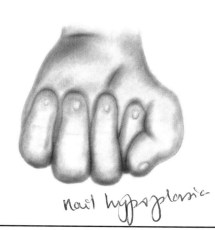

Nail hypoplasia

Fetal hydantoin syndrome is due to fetal exposure to phenytoin. It is synonymous with phenytoin embryopathy or Dilantin embryopathy

The drawings depict the following features:

- Microcephaly
- Broad nasal bridge,
- Low hairline,
- Short neck,
- Hypertelorism,
- Low set ears,
- Epicanthal folds,
- Coarse scalp hair

Additional findings could include :

- Large anterior fontanelle
- Ptosis
- Coloboma
- Broad alveolar ridge
- Cleft lip/palate
- Small or absent nails
- Hypoplasia of distal phalanges
- Dislocated hip

Hand findings would include

- Palmar crease
- Digital thumb

Fetal Valproate Syndrome

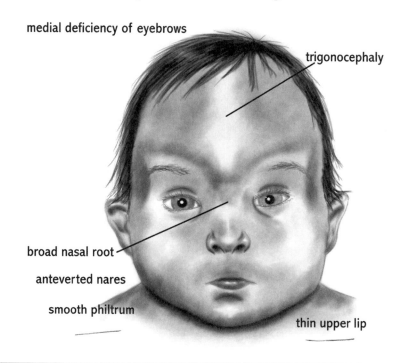

medial deficiency of eyebrows

trigonocephaly

broad nasal root

anteverted nares

smooth philtrum

thin upper lip

Marfan Syndrome

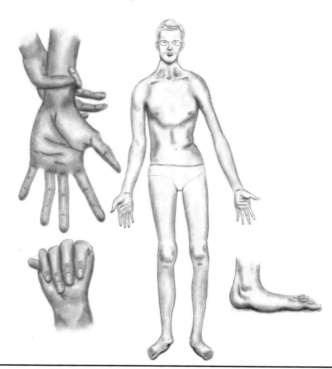

©Medhumor Medical Publications, LLC

This drawing includes the following features of Marfan syndrome:

- Long and narrow face
- Myopia (patient is wearing glasses)
- Pectus carinatum (excavatum also common)
- Arms and legs unusually long in proportion to torso
- Reduced extension of the elbows (<170°)
- Scoliosis greater than 20°
- Flat feet.
- Arachnodactyly: elongated fingers and toes

Two simple maneuvers demonstrate arachnodactyly:

- **Wrist sign:** distal phalanges of first and fifth digits of one hand overlap when wrapped around opposite wrist
- **Thumb sign**: thumb, when completely opposed within clenched hand, projects beyond ulnar border

INSIDER TIPS

Medical historians believe that Abraham Lincoln had many features of Marfan Syndrome.
See the following link for some interesting information on this subject:
http://www.doctorzebra.com/prez/g16.htm

Potters Facies

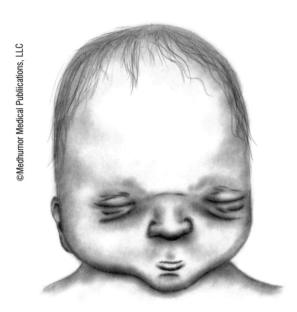

©Medhumor Medical Publications, LLC

The illustration demonstrates the typical Potter's Facie including the prominent infraorbital folds

This is a direct result of oligohydramnios which results from the absence of normal functioning kidneys.

The facial deformation is due to constraint in utero.

Prune Belly Eagle

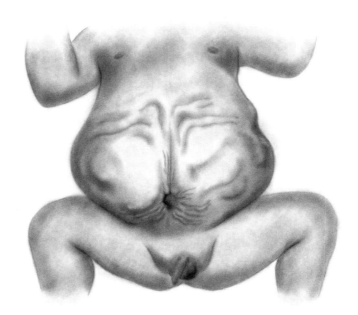

The drawing depicts the deficient abdominal musculature and bilateral cryptorchidism

Prune belly syndrome is also associated with

- Renal hypoplasia
- Oligohydramnios
- Urinary tract malformation

Pseudohypoparathyroidism
(Albright Hereditary Osteodystrophy)

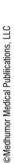

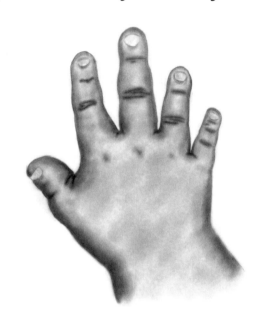

The illustration demonstrates the following:

- Brachydactyly with shortening of third through fifth metacarpals and distal phalanx of thumb
- Dimples may replace knuckles on affected fingers
- Short stature
- Round face

William Syndrome

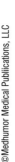

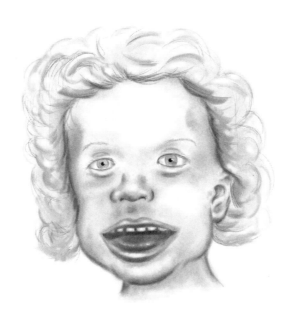

The facial features depicted in the drawing include:

- Broad forehead
- Stellate irides[1]
- Periorbital fullness
- Short upturned nose
- Flat nasal bridge
- Long philtrum
- Flat malar area
- Wide mouth with full lips
- Widely spaced teeth
- Micrognathia.

The prototypical facial features are often termed "Elfin facies". This is now considered a derogatory term. However we have included it in case the term is used on the exam in the descriptive history.

William syndrome is also associated with strabismus which is not included in the drawing.

---

[1] This term refers to the prominent "starburst" or white lacy pattern of the iris.

GI

Upper GI Series (Barium Swallow)

©Medhumor Medical Publications, LLC

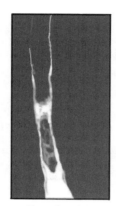

GERD

- Barium fills esophagus
- Wide gastro-esophageal jct

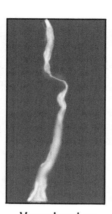

Esophagitis

- Irregular mucosa
- Superficial erosions or ulcerations
- Small barium streaks, dots, or outpouchings

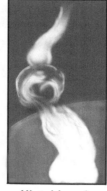

Vascular ring

- Narrowing or pinching of esophagus

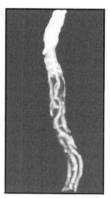

Hiatal hernia

- Gastric mucosa above diaphragm
- Note gastric folds or barium streaks

Esophageal varices

- Serpiginous thickening of longitudinal folds
- Tortuous longitudinal filling defects
- Hint: portal HTN or splenomegaly

DEFINITION

GERD (Gastroesophageal Reflux) is the reflux of gastric contents into the esophagus usually due to relaxation of the esophageal sphincter. This is usually a temporary condition that infants outgrow.

LOOK FOR

Along with the typical picture of a barium swallow the history includes and infant "**spits up**" after feeding or one that "**chokes**" "**gag**s" or "**vomits**" a short while after feeding. [1]

INSIDER TIPS

If the reflux results in vagal nerve stimulation they may also describe *apnea, bradycardia,* or even *cyanosis* and *pallor.*

The signs and symptoms of **hiatal hernia** are often very similar to those of GERD, note the difference in the barium swallow in order to better differentiate them on the exam.

Vascular Ring will often present as projectile vomiting in a newborn along with the typical barium swallow illustrated.

---

[1] The quotes are deliberate since these will often be terms described by parents and are often placed in quotes in the question.

Tracheoesophageal Fistula (TEF)

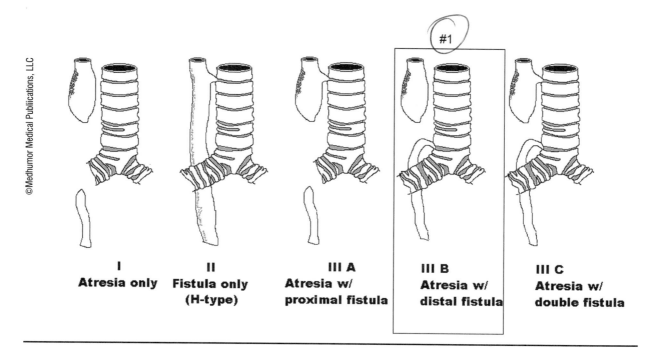

©Medhumor Medical Publications, LLC

I
Atresia only

II
Fistula only (H-type)

III A
Atresia w/ proximal fistula

III B
Atresia w/ distal fistula

III C
Atresia w/ double fistula

 The most common type of TE Fistula is *proximal esophageal atresia* with fistula connecting the distal esophagus to the trachea.

A common presentation of the H type fistula would be a 3 month old with a recurrent wheeze. Additional findings would include *gagging accumulation of mucus as well as saliva.*

In extreme cases the history can also include *cyanosis, vomiting,* as well as *aspiration pneumonia.*

Polyhydramnios may be a part of the prenatal history.

The most common type of TE Fistula is Type III B shown which includes esophageal atresia with a fistula connecting the distal esophageal remnant to the trachea.

The presentation of this most common form includes the accumulation of secretions as described above as well as the inability to pass a gastric tube [2] with the coiled tube in the blind esophageal pouch visible on x-ray.

---

[2] Of course we are assuming this is being performed by somebody who is otherwise skilled enough to pass the NG tube successfully.

LOOK FOR

In fact this is the picture they may present on the exam. This x-ray combined with the typical history should make this an easy slam dunk on the exam.

Meconium Ileus

Multiple bowel loops

Microcolon

Inspissated meconium w/ soap-bubble appearance

Hint: think of cystic fibrosis

©Medhumor Medical Publications, LLC

LOOK FOR

On abdominal plain film or CXR that include the abdomen, look for *multiple loops of bowel*, *microcolon soap-bubble appearance* consisting of *inspissated stool.*

MNEMONIC

When you are presented with a pictorial demonstrating meconium ileus, **cystic fibrosis** should come to mind.

Intestinal Malrotation & Valvulus

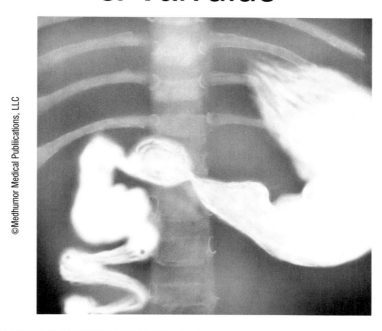

©Medhumor Medical Publications, LLC

In a normal upper GI the duodenum crosses midline, creating a "C-loop" appearance. This is missing in malrotation and volvulus.

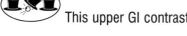

This upper GI contrast study illustrated above shows volvulus.

Important features of the study include:

- The proximal duodenum is dilated with a spiral or "corkscrew" appearance distally.
- The duodenal –Jejunal junction is misplaced to the right of midline.

Newborns present with bilious vomiting and feeding intolerance. Older children present more insidiously.

Heme, Onc

Ewing Sarcoma

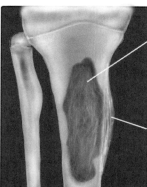

©Medhumor Medical Publications, LLC

Long, medullary, lytic lesion most common

May extend into soft-tissue

Periosteal reaction
-"Onion-skin" appearance #1
-"Sunburst" pattern less common

diaphysis – ES
metaphysis – OS

-#2 bone tumor in kids, but most lethal
-Metaphysis/diaphysis of long bones
-Risk factors: adolescent, WHITE, male (Hint: think of JR Ewing)

With Ewing Sarcoma they will either describe or show a lesion in one of the long bones with *periosteal reaction extending into soft tissue*. This will often be *described* as **onion skin pattern**.

This will often be described in an *adolescent white male*. Ewing sarcoma also typically involves the axial skeleton and the lesion is primarily *lytic*.

Ewing sarcoma is primarily lytic.[1]
Osteogenic sarcoma is primarily *sclerotic*.
Osteogenic Sarcoma is more common than Ewing Sarcoma.

---

[1] In osteogenic sarcoma it can be a combination of lytic and sclerotic lesions however if pressed to make a choice lytic would be the correct choice.

Ewing and Osteogenic Sarcoma / The fine Differences

	Ewing	Osteogenic Sarcoma
X-ray	Onion Picture somebody peeling onions saying " EEEWing" as tears run down their eyes.	Sunburst
Presentation	Can present with **systemic symptoms** such as fatigue, fever and weight loss, along with pain and decreased range of motion.	*Localized pain* and swelling. Often the history will include the description of a minor trauma. This will often throw you off during the exam. Pain that is beyond the norm for the level of injury is a classic presentation of osteogenic sarcoma especially on the boards.

Osteogenic Sarcoma
(Osteosarcoma)

"Moth-eaten appearance" = lesion usually both sclerotic and lytic

Periosteal reaction may produce:
1. Codman triangle = elevation
2. Sunburst pattern = spiculation

Destruction of bone and cortex w/ extension into soft tissue

Variable soft-tissue calcification

©Medhumor Medical Publications, LLC

-#1 bone tumor in kids
-Ends of humerus & femur most common
-Risk factors: adolescent male
-Metastasizes early to lungs & other bones

LOOK FOR

They will often describe or show a moth eaten appearance which is consistent with a combination of sclerotic and lytic lesions. The periosteal reaction will result in

- **Codman Triangle**
- **Sunburst appearance**

LOOK FOR

Look for the destruction of bone and cortex with extension into soft-tissue along with soft tissue calcification.

It typically presents in adolescent males involving the long bones of the arm and legs, also known as the humerus and femur in orthopedic and anatomy circles.

INSIDER TIPS

Osteogenic sarcoma *metastasizes* to other *bones* and to the *lungs*.

Osteogenic Osteoma

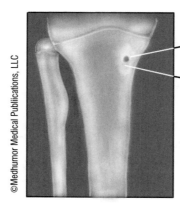

Round nidus < 2 cm

Intense periosteal blastic bone response

-Cortex of long bones most common
-Risk factors: white, male
-Pain at night, relieved w/ NSAIDs

Osteoid osteoma is a benign tumor, pain mostly at night relieved by aspirin or NSAID, typically involving long bones especially the tibia or femur

Treatment is surgical excision

Rhabdomyosarcoma
aka "Sarcoma Botryoides" when vaginal

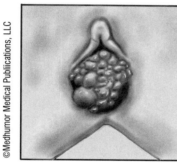

- #1 soft-tissue sarcoma in kids
- Aggressive, highly malignant tumor
- Head/neck, urogenital tract, extremities
- Vagina: protruding polypoid mass "bunch of grapes"

Bimodal incidence:
1st peak 2-5 y/o
2nd peak adolescence

Risk factors:
- Neurofibromatosis
- Beckwith-Wiedemann syndrome
- Radiation

©Medhumor Medical Publications, LLC

Sarcoma botryoides is a form of rhabdomyosarcoma in the vaginal area frequently appearing in the illustration part of the board exam as a protruding polypoid mass.

In addition rhabdomyosarcoma can also be seen in the *head neck and the extremities.*

Sarcoma botryoides will typically be described in a child age 2-5 or in an adolescent.

Rhabdomyosarcoma is associated with **neurofibromatosis, Beckwith-Wiedemann syndrome, and a history of radiation exposure.**

Neonatology

Cephalohematoma
vs Caput Succedaneum

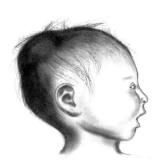 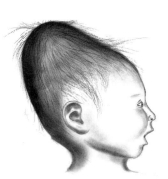

- SubPeriosteal Hemorrhage
- Limited by sutures
  -- LH = Lump on Head
- Weeks to months resolve
  -- May calcify
- Due to birth trauma
  -- Vacuum extraction #1

- SubQ edema
- CS = Crosses Sutures
- Few days to resolve
- Normal process
- "Conehead" appearance

venous stasis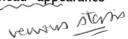

	Caput succedaneum	**Cephalohematoma**
Suture Lines	Crosses the suture lines	Localized does *not* cross the suture lines
Appearance	Cone head appearance	Discolored, firm and tense. Can be associated with non depressed skull fracture
When	Part of normal birth process. Appears at the time of delivery	During *birth trauma* i.e. vacuum or forceps extraction. Appears hours after birth
Resolves	Within days	Takes *2 -12 weeks* to resolve

Change the name to Cap **SucCONE-DAYseum** to remember the association of caput succedaneum.

Gastroschisis

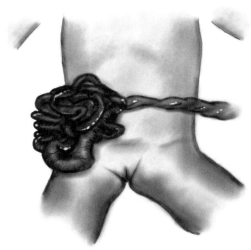

Abdominal viscera exposed

Herniation through abdominal wall
- uniform in size (5 cm)
- usually to RIGHT of umbilical cord

Inflamed intestine: thick, edematous, shortened, matted loops w/ surface exudate (peel)

Complications: malabsorption, bowel necrosis

Risk factors:
- mother young w/ low gravity
- first-born child
- prematurity
- IUGR

Hint: Imagine a necrotic, twisted letter "G" poking out of belly

---

The abdominal viscera is exposed and *not covered by a membrane* .

Typically herniated to the *right of the umbilicus with the umbilicus remaining intact*

Maternal history usually, young, low gravity, first born, typically premature with IUGR

Twisted letter G to the right of the umbilicus

Remember IV fluid hydration is important prior to surgery.

Omphalocele is associated with

    1) The defect through the midline of the umbilicus.

    2) The protruding bowel is covered with peritoneum

Omphalocele is associated with Beckwith-Wiedemann Syndrome as well as Edward Syndrome and myelomeningocele.

Gastroschisis:

- Is located to the right of the umbilicus. Bowel contents are exposed at the time of delivery.
- The umbilical cord is intact.

Brachial Plexus Injury

Erb palsy

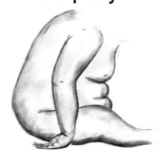

Klumpke palsy

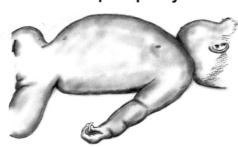

- C5, C6, & C7 = upper plexus
- Limply adducted and internally rotated arm w/ pronated forearm
- "Waiter's tip" posture
- Grasp reflex preserved
- Complication: diaphragmatic paralysis

newer praxic

Hint: Herb the Waiter

- C7, C8, & T1 = lower plexus
- Upper arm unaffected
- Absent grasp reflex
- "Clawhand" deformity
- Complication: Horner syndrome (miosis, ptosis, anhydrosis)

Hint: Klumpke the Klaw

poor prognosis

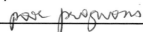

Being able to distinguish these two birth related brachial plexus injuries is worthy of your time and at least one point on the exam!

- Erb palsy involves C5, 6. Recognizing the picture is easy since it is a waiter tip position remembered as the waiter receiving an "herb" instead of money.
- Klumpke palsy involved C7, C8 and T1. Primarily lower arm paralysis with tendon reflexes intact but poor grasping reflex due to wasting of intrinsic muscles of the hand.

- In *Erb palsy* grip reflex is often *preserved*.
- In *Klumpke* it is *not preserved*.
- Diaphragmatic paralysis is often an associated finding with Erb Palsy.

Horner Syndrome (ptosis, anhidrosis and miosis) is associated with Klumpke Palsy

Remember the waiter can still grip his tip but Klumpke is clumsy and therefore cannot. Hold on. Eye problems (Horner syndrome) would occur if somebody flung a "Klumpke" of sand in your eye. You can remember that diaphragmatic hernia is associated with Erb Palsy when you consider the waiter has his "breath taken away" from the shock of receiving an herb instead of a cash tip.

Cytomegalovirus vs Toxoplasmosis

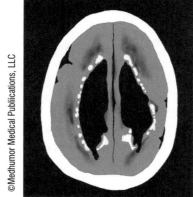

©Medhumor Medical Publications, LLC

Cytomegalovirus (CMV)
-Calcifications CENTRAL (periventricular)
-Lissencephaly, polymicrogyria
-Ventricular dilatation
-Cerebellar hypoplasia

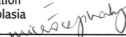
microcephaly

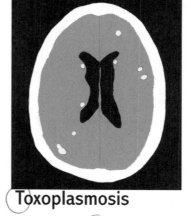

Toxoplasmosis
-Calcifications THROUGHOUT (periventricular, basal ganglia, cerebral cortex
-Hydrocephalus

Cytomegalovirus

- The calcification in cytomegalovirus is central or periventricular.
- In addition look for cerebellar hypoplasia and ventricular dilatation.

Toxoplasmosis

- The calcifications are throughout including periventricular, basal ganglia, cerebral cortex.
- In addition, look for hydrocephalus.

It is easy to remember that cytomegalovirus calcifications are central since **c**ytomegalovirus and **c**entral both start with **C**. Therefore, it is easy to remember that **T**oxoplasmosis and **t**hroughout both start with a **T**.

Choanal Atresia

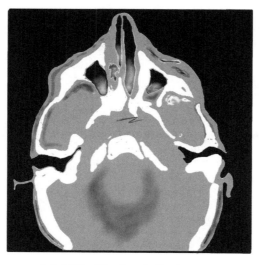

Axial CT with classic features:
- Widening of posterior septum
- "Funneling" of nasal airway
- Mucus in nasal cavities
- Bony > membranous

Choanal Atresia is diagnosed by CT scan therefore consider this diagnosis especially if presented with a head CT of a neonate.

The classic findings on head CT are

- Widening of the posterior septum
- Funneling of the nasal airway
- Mucous in the nasal cavities

Choanal Atresia comes in 2 varieties
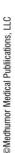
1. Bony
2. Membranous

Bony is seen more frequently than membranous. At least more frequently in the reality based clinical world, remember the boards are different where zebras plow the fields and are the thoroughbreds at the track.

Since neonates are obligate nasal breathers, the classic history is of an infant who becomes *cyanotic during feedings* which is alleviated when the infant cries.

The diagnosis is then confirmed when a nasal catheter cannot be passed.

This would not apply with *unilateral* choanal atresia.

Choanal Atresia can be associated with CHARGE syndrome which is an acronym for

> **C**oloboma
> **H**eart defects
> **A**tresia (Choanal Atresia our featured disorder on this page)
> **R**etarded (Growth retardation)
> **G** GU problems
> **E**ar – hearing loss

Spina Bifida

Meningomyelocele

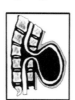

- Severest form
- Spinal cord and meninges protrude through defect

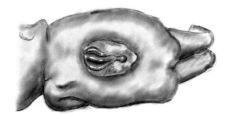

Spina bifida occulta

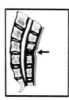

- Mildest form
- Vertebral defect
- Dimple or hairy patch in overlying skin

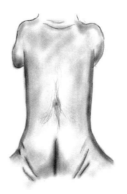

©Medhumor Medical Publications, LLC

Congenital Syphilis

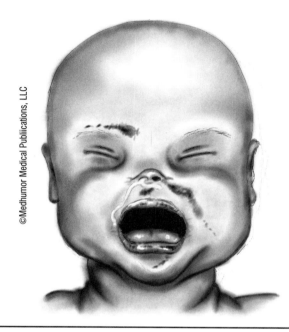

©Medhumor Medical Publications, LLC

EARLY
- "SNUFFLES" = chronic rhinitis/coryza, often mucopurolent +/- blood
- SPLENOMEGALY > hepatomegaly
- bullae on hands and feet
- nasty umbilical cord

LATE
- skin infiltration: diffusely firm & shiny, pink-red then coppery-brown
- "RHAGADES" = fine linear fissures & mucous patches near nose, mouth, anus
- Hutchinson teeth: notched, widely spaced, & peg shaped
- Mulberry Molar: abnormal cusp & enamel
- Saddle nose

BONE-US: X-ray showing "moth-eaten" distal ends of long bones or Sabre shins

Symptoms often delayed weeks to months

Congenital syphilis may not present until a few weeks after birth.

Facial features included in the drawing includes:

- "Snuffles": Profuse, mucopurulent blood-tinged nasal discharge
- Mucocutaneous patches and ulcerations at the mouth

Additional findings would include mucocutaneous patches and ulcerations around the anus, vulva, or scrotum.

Congenital Ptosis

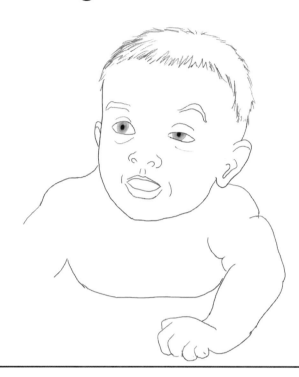

©Medhumor Medical Publications, LLC

DEFINITION Congenital ptosis is due to dysgenesis of the levator palpebrae superioris. This results in dysfunction of the levator extraocular muscle.

INSIDER TIPS In addition to being expected to recognize this you are expected to know that obstruction of visual field can lead to permanent loss of vision (amblyopia) unless corrected by age 8 years

Hutchinson Teeth
vs Dental Caries

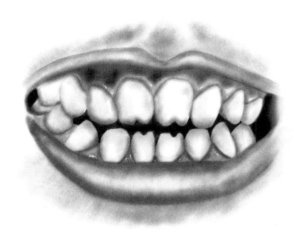

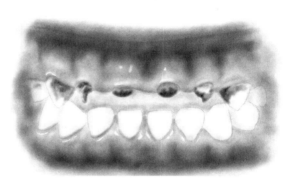

©Medhumor Medical Publications, LLC

    Please note these similar drawings and how they differ. Dental caries will clearly depict the dark spots of caries and the shape of the teeth typical of bottle fed caries. This is quite different in appearance than Hutchinson teeth associated with congenital syphilis.

In addition note:

Hutchinson teeth are small and widely spaced with pegged lateral incisors and notched central incisors. Only the permanent teeth are affected.

Baby bottle tooth decay (early childhood caries) is only seen in infants and toddlers. Top four front teeth most affected. May affect alignment of permanent teeth.

Ophthalmology

Esotropia vs Pseudoesotropia

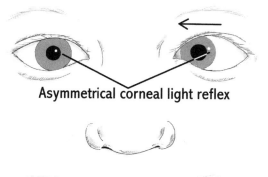

Asymmetrical corneal light reflex

- TRUE ESOTROPIA
  -- Large esodeviation = "crossed eyes"
  -- Congenital, acquired, or accomodative
  -- Deviation worsens when child tired = "lazy eye"
  -- Left untreated, can lead to amblyopia (decreased vision

- Transient strabismus: normal up to age 3 months ✈ ✈

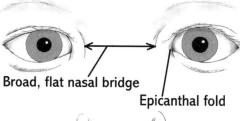

Broad, flat nasal bridge

Epicanthal fold

- PSEUDOESOTROPIA
  -- Common up to age 4 years
  -- Medial (nasal) sclera partially covered
  -- Symmetric corneal light reflex

Pseudoesotropia

Two key findings differentiating pseudo from esotropia is the equal corneal reflexes seen in pseudo-esotropia and partial covering of the nasal/medial sclera in pseudo-esotropia.

Cataract

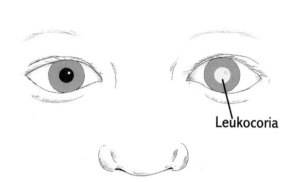

©Medhumor Medical Publications, LLC

Leukocoria

LOOK FOR

The pupil's size will be equal and they will either describe or show leukocoria. ✓

Cataracts in an infant can be seen with Rubella, Galactosemia, and Down syndrome.

INSIDER TIPS

Watch for *nystagmus* and/or other visual disturbances in the history to help solidify this as the correct answer.

INSIDER TIPS

If congenital cataracts are diagnosed or a red reflex is absent an ophthalmology[1] consult should be made immediately. It is one of the rare cases where calling a specialist will be the correct answer on the boards.

INSIDER TIPS

Cataracts are associated with several metabolic disorders including galactosemia, diabetes melitis, and Lowe syndrome. Galactosemia in particular is a board favorite.

---

[1] Hopefully you can spell ophthalmology correctly. It is frequently spelled incorrectly even in hospitals. But if you are reading this footnote, you do not have to know how to spell on the exam so you can stop reading this tangential comment and get back to studying.

Normal Fundus

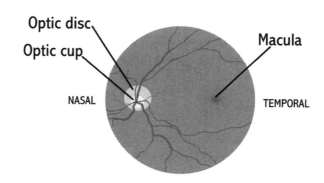

It is important to keep in mind the findings of a normal funduscopic exam.

Glaucoma

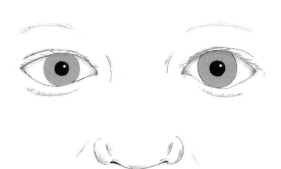

- Different-sized eyes (affected eye larger)
- Corneal opacity or clouding
- Irregular corneal light reflex or dull red reflex
- Pain, photophobia, & tearing

Look for an irregular corneal light reflex or the description of a dull red reflex.

An increased corneal diameter will almost always be demonstrated

Look for a history or pain, and tearing

Congenital Glaucoma

Excessive tearing, photophobia large cornea diameter, white or red eye.

Retinoblastoma

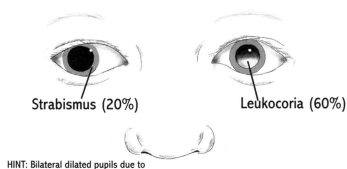

Strabismus (20%)   Leukocoria (60%)

HINT: Bilateral dilated pupils due to
ophthalmologic dilation

©Medhumor Medical Publications, LLC

Key findings with retinoblastoma are

- Leukocoria and strabismus

Watch for bilateral mydriasis (dilated eyes) which would be iatrogenic since that is what eye doctors also known as ophthalmologists do

The absence of a red reflex is an important finding

Orthopaedics

Rickets

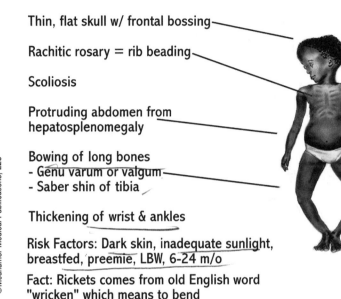

Thin, flat skull w/ frontal bossing

Rachitic rosary = rib beading

Scoliosis

Protruding abdomen from hepatosplenomegaly

Bowing of long bones
- Genu varum or valgum
- Saber shin of tibia

Thickening of wrist & ankles

Risk Factors: Dark skin, inadequate sunlight, breastfed, preemie, LBW, 6-24 m/o

Fact: Rickets comes from old English word "wricken" which means to bend

Radiologic findings:
- May precede clinical manifestations
- Widening of physes
- Irregular "frayed" metaphyseal margins
- Splayed, cupped metaphyses
- Osteopenia
- Bowing of extremities

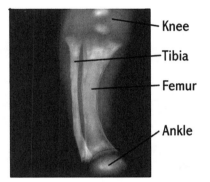

- Knee
- Tibia
- Femur
- Ankle

©Medhumor Medical Publications, LLC

Signs of Rickets on **Physical Exam**

It is best to try to remember the signs of rickets literally from head to toe, since they can show you any one of these in isolation on the exam.

Head – Frontal Bossing   *Craniotabes*

Chest - Rachitic rosary, rib beading. They might show this on x-ray

Back - Scoliosis

Abdomen - Protruding abdomen secondary to hepatomegaly

Long bones:

- Bowing of long bones-
- Thickening of wrists and ankles

Signs of Rickets **x-ray studies**

They will always show at least one x-ray finding of rickets on the exam, knowing these cold will get you at least one point on the exam.

 The x-ray findings may precede any clinical manifestations, therefore do not be thrown by this if they show you any of the typical x-ray findings of rickets in what you believe is a "normal" child.

The *radiological findings* include:

- Widening of the physes
- Frayed metaphyseal margins
- Cupped metaphyses
- Osteopenia
- Bowing of the extremities

This is one of the rear cases where breast feeding can be a negative.

Metaphyseal Fracture
("bucket handle" or "corner" fracture)

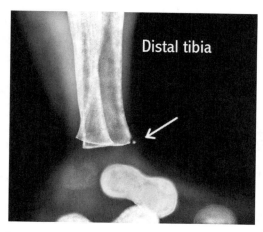

Distal tibia

©Medhumor Medical Publications, LLC

- SPECIFIC for abuse (diagnostic)
- Knee, ankle, shoulder
- Planar fracture through growth plate
due to shearing effect of shaking

The metaphyseal bucket handle fracture is a result of shearing forces causing a planar fracture through the growth plate.

Metaphyseal fractures are diagnostic for child abuse

They could insert the word 'buckle fracture" to throw you off. Read the words/questions carefully.

Scheuermann Kyphosis

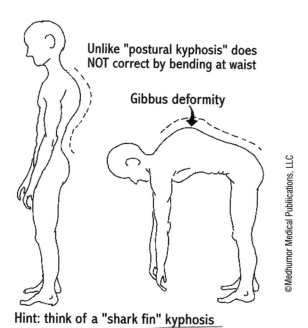

Unlike "postural kyphosis" does NOT correct by bending at waist

Gibbus deformity

©Medhumor Medical Publications, LLC

Hint: think of a "shark fin" kyphosis

Talipes Equinovarus

(Clubfoot)

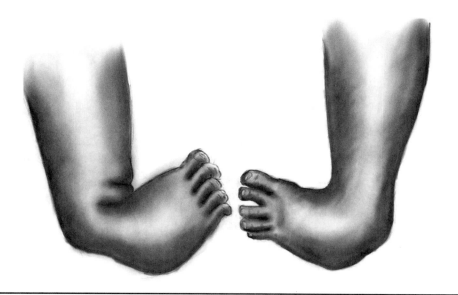

The drawing depicts the heel turned inward and the foot plantar flexed typical of talipes equinovarus.

These findings are noted at birth, the foot turns inward and downward, resisting realignment.

 This is also known as club foot deformity

Abdominal Studies

Normal IVP

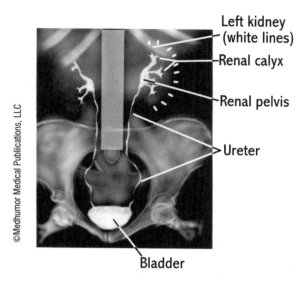

Left kidney
(white lines)

Renal calyx

Renal pelvis

Ureter

Bladder

©Medhumor Medical Publications, LLC

Despite the decreasing use of IVP as a diagnostic tool it could still make an appearance on the exam.

Therefore it is important that you be able to identify the normal components of an IVP in the absence of renal pathology.

Duplication of Urinary Collecting System

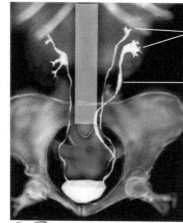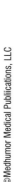

Duplicated collecting system

Vesicoureteral reflux in ureter from lower pole

©Medhumor Medical Publications, LLC

30% bilateral, many variations

Risk of: recurrent UTI or hydronephrosis

Duplication of the urinary collecting system on IVP in addition to duplicated collecting system will also show vesicoureteral reflux in the ureter from the lower pole.

INSIDER TIPS

Keep in mind the high risk for and history of UTI and hydronephrosis

---

Wilms Tumor - IVP

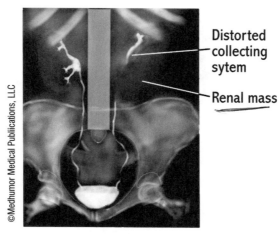

Distorted collecting sytem

Renal mass

Tip: Look for hematuria, hypertension, aniridia, or hemihypertrophy

---

Wilms tumor on IVP will feature a distorted collecting system as well as a renal mass.

Wilms tumor can also be referred to as nephroblastoma, as one of the choices. At casual glance this can be mistaken for the word neuroblastoma. It would be a pity to get an easy question wrong on such a careless error.

The clinical description will include, hematuria, hypertension, hemihypertrophy and aniridia.

4 H's of Wilms tumor.

WAGR

Hematuria, **h**ypertension, **h**emihypertrophy, and **h**ijacked iris (aniridia)

Wilms Tumor - CT

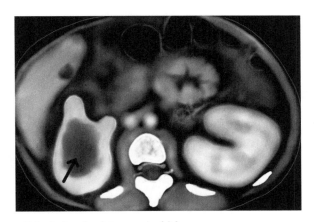

©Medhumor Medical Publications, LLC

- #1 abdominal tumor in kids
- #1 presentation: asymptomatic abdominal mass
- Unilateral > bilateral
- Typical case: 3 y/o white +/- abdominal pain

Tip: Look for hematuria, hypertension, aniridia, or hemihypertrophy

As noted in the IVP pictorial the tumor is " intra-renal"

 Wilms tumor presents as an *asymptomatic* abdominal mass.

Neuroblastoma

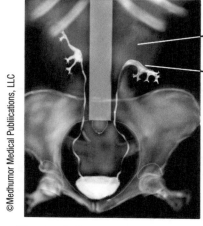

Extrarenal mass

"Drooping lily" sign from downward displacement of collecting system

©Medhumor Medical Publications, LLC

Tip: Look for metastases and remote effects (proptosis, ataxia, or opsomyoclonus)

In neuroblastoma, there is an external mass impinging on the kidney.

Therefore the collecting system is pushed down resulting in the drooping lily sign

They may also show or describe other signs such as metastases and other associations with neuroblastoma such as proptosis, ataxia and opsomyoclonus).

Differences between Neuroblastoma and Wilms Tumor

Both Wilms tumor and Neuroblastoma are abdominal masses with a lot in common. However it is the subtle differences in the imaging studies and text that will allow you slam dunk a correct answer.

Table 1 below outlines the differences and similarities

Wilms V.S. neuroblastoma

Both Neuroblastoma and Wilms Tumor present as abdominal masses, fever and weight loss. They are both diagnosed with a combination of Ultrasound, CT scan and biopsy

However the differences outlined below are the important points to learn and review.

Table 1

	Neuroblastoma	Wilms Tumor
Physical Findings	Abdominal Mass Hypertension Opsoclonus[1] Myoclonus Raccoon eyes	Abdominal and *flank* mass Hemihypertrophy Aniridia Additional less well known findings in Wilms tumor include Hypospadias and one kidney
Lab Findings	Elevated catecholamines in urine[2]	Hematuria
Imaging Studies	Derives from the adrenals or sympathetic nerve chain and *does* cross the midline MIBG Scan is positive[3]	Derives from the kidney and does not cross the midline on imaging studies MIBG Scan is negative

PERIL
WARNING   The raccoon eyes or periorbital ecchymosis are often mistaken for physical abuse a point taken advantage of on the boards. Watch for the implication of abuse in a child with raccoon eyes who has all of the other hallmarks of neuroblastoma.

---

[1] Consider myoclonus and opsoclonus to be the equivalent of dancing feet and eyes respectively.

[2] i.e. homovanillic and vanillylmandelic acids

[3] MIBG (Iodine-131-Meta-Iodobenzylguanidine) Scintiscan the radioisotope is taken up by adrenal and sympathetic secreting tissue.

Renal Ectopia

Both kidneys on right side

Ureteropelvic junction obstruction common

Left ureter crosses over

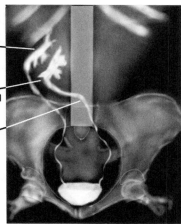

©Medhumor Medical Publications, LLC

Look for: **Klippel-Feil syndrome**

The common features seen with renal ectopia are *both kidneys on the right side, ureteropelvic obstruction with the left ureter crossing over.*

It is associated with Klippel-Feil syndrome   *vertebral anomalies*

Vesicoureteral Reflux

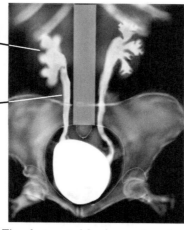

Dilated pelvis
and calyces

Dilated ureter

©Medhumor Medical Publications, LLC

Tip: Antenatal hydronephrosis or
postnatal UTI

Look for reflux nephropathy: HTN
and renal failure

Vesicoureteral reflux on IVP features *dilated pelvis and calyces and dilated ureter*.

Look for prenatal hydronephrosis and post natal UTI

Reflux nephropathy includes hypertensin and renal failure

Uretero-Pelvic Junction (UPJ) Obstruction

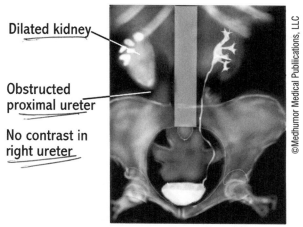

Dilated kidney

Obstructed proximal ureter

No contrast in right ureter

©Medhumor Medical Publiications, LLC

#1 cause of upper tract obstruction in kids

Risk of: hydronephrosis, poor renal function, recurrent UTIs

If they were to throw you an IVP UVP obstruction would be in your differential

In the IVP look for dilated kidney, obstructed proximal ureter, no contrast in the right ureter.

Number 1 cause of upper tract obstruction in children

UVP obstruction leaves patients at risk for pyelonephritis and recurrent UTI's

---

Brain Imaging

Brain Abscess

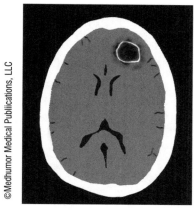

©Medhumor Medical Publications, LLC

Round or oval lesion with enhancing rim and surrounding edema

Differential = tumor & resolving hematoma

A brain abscess on head CT will be demonstrated as **round dark oval with enhancing rim** (white) with surrounding edema.

The CT of a tumor and a resolving hematoma look very similar. It is on the basis of the presenting history that you will be able to differentiate the two.

Brain Tumor

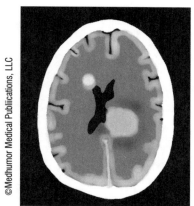

CT scan of supratentorial tumor:
malignant glioblastoma
- Hyperdense mass in bilateral
basal ganglia ✓
- Look for calcification ✓

Supratentorial Brain Tumor

An example of a supratentorial brain tumor would be a malignant glioblastoma.

 Look for bilateral hyperdense mass in the basal ganglia.

 Calcification would be an important factor in making this diagnosis in the exam.

Posterior Fossa Medulloblastoma

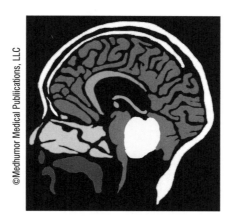

©Medhumor Medical Publications, LLC

Contrast MRI scan showing midline,
posterior-fossa medulloblastoma
- Contrast-enhancing 4th ventricle mass
- Hydrocephalus

Posterior Fossa Medulloblastoma

If a Posterior fossa tumor is suspected the correct diagnostic study to order is a *contrast MRI.*

The contrast MRI study will demonstrate a contrast enhancing 4th ventricle mass as well as hydrocephalus.

Dandy-Walker Malformation

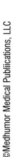
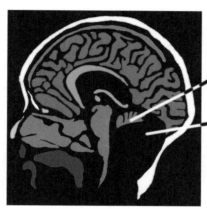

©Medhumor Medical Publications, LLC

MRI showing TRIAD of findings:

1. Partial/complete agenesis of cerebellar vermis

2. Cystic dilatation of 4th ventricle

3. Enlarged posterior fossa
Hydrocephalus = common complication

Look for a Brain MRI with the following findings:

Dandy Walker Malformation Triad

1) Partial or complete agenesis of the Cerebellar Vermis.
2) Cystic Dilatation of the 4th Ventricle.
3) Enlarged Posterior Fossa.

Hydrocephalus is a common complication or Dandy Walker Malformation.

Subdural Hematoma vs Epidural Hematoma

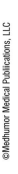

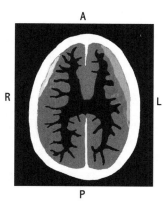

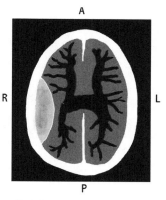

Subdural hematomas
- Venous in origin
- Hyperdense (white) acute on R
- Isodense (gray) subacute on L
- Crescent shaped
- Bilateral common in infants
- Parietal region #1

Epidural hematoma
- Arterial in origin
- Biconvex or lens-shaped hyperdense area
- Blood between skull and dura
- Temporal region #1
- Crosses dural attachments, not sutures
- #1 cause = trauma (usually blunt)

Subdural hematomas are venous in origin.

Look for hyperdense, white crescent shaped, usually in the parietal region.

Subdural hematomas can be bilateral in infants.

Epidural hematomas are arterial in origin.

In Epidural hematomas look for a biconcave or lens shaped hyperdense area which represents blood between the skull and the dura.

The temporal region is the typical area involvement in Epidural hematomas (Temporal).

In Epidural hematomas the bleeding crosses the dural attachments not the suture lines.

The usual cause of Epidural hematomas is trauma. 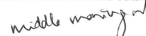 middle meningeal

Achondroplasia Cervicomedullary Compression

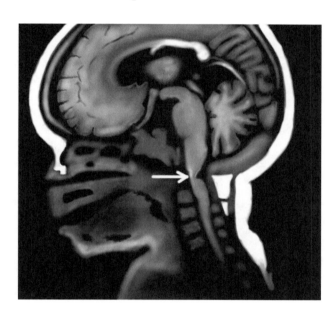

©Medhumor Medical Publications, LLC

The following features are depicted in the drawing of achondroplasia cervicomedullary compression

- Narrowing at foramen magnum with compression of the cervicomedullary junction
- The posterior fossa is somewhat small appearing

Cerebellar Brain Tumor

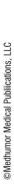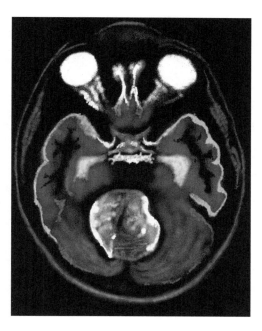

©Medhumor Medical Publications, LLC

 The brain MRI depicted shows a solid, heterogeneous, midline cerebellar mass

The heterogeneity probably results from the cysts and calcification

The specific tumor demonstrated is a medulloblastoma, the #1 malignant brain tumor in children

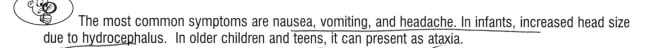 The most common symptoms are nausea, vomiting, and headache. In infants, increased head size due to hydrocephalus. In older children and teens, it can present as ataxia.

The differential diagnosis of cerebellar tumors include: astrocytoma (usually pilocytic), ependymoma and posterior fossa cyst.

Tuberous Sclerosis Complex

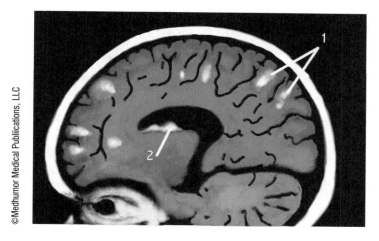

©Medhumor Medical Publications, LLC

1. Cortical tubers
2. Subependymal nodules (SENs)

The drawing of the MRI depicting tuberous sclerosis included the following

Sagittal view shows:

1. **Cortical tubers:** hyperintense (white) lesions in cerebral cortex. These are the most characteristic lesion of TS.

2. **Subependymal nodules:** found on wall of lateral ventricles, usually near Foramen of Monroe. These are often described as "candle drippings". .

Both cortical tubers and subependymal nodules are considered hamartomas and major criteria for diagnosis.

Chest Films

Esophageal Coin

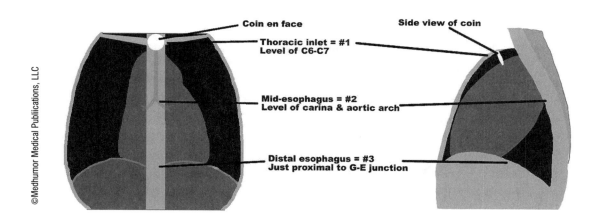

Coin en face

Side view of coin

Thoracic inlet = #1
Level of C6-C7

Mid-esophagus = #2
Level of carina & aortic arch

Distal esophagus = #3
Just proximal to G-E junction

©Medhumor Medical Publications, LLC

When the coin is in the esophagus you will see the coin face on in the PA film

You will see the coin's edge on the lateral film

Note on the film where the mid esophagus is and where the distal esophagus is.

Phrenic Nerve Paralysis

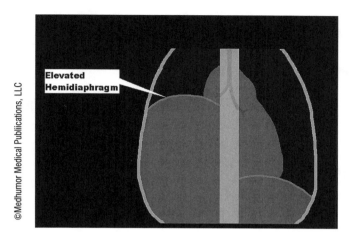

Look for elevated hemi-diaphragm

Can be seen with Erb's Palsy

Diaphragmatic Hernia

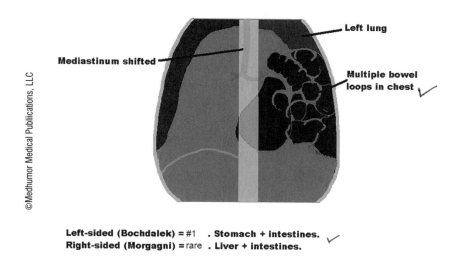

Diaphragmatic Hernia usually involves the left lung

Look for multiple bowel loops in the left chest as well as a mediastinal shift to the right

Duodenal Atresia

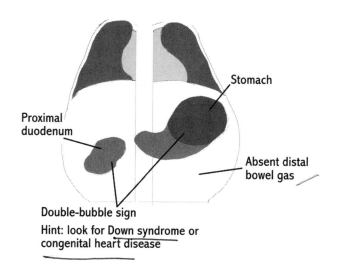

©Medhumor Medical Publications, LLC

Stomach

Proximal duodenum

Absent distal bowel gas

Double-bubble sign

Hint: look for Down syndrome or congenital heart disease

The classic sign on x-ray is the double bubble sign.

Duodenal atresia t is associated with Down syndrome and/or congential heart disease, therefore look for this presented in the history

Look for the absence of distal bowel gas.

Aspiration Pneumonia

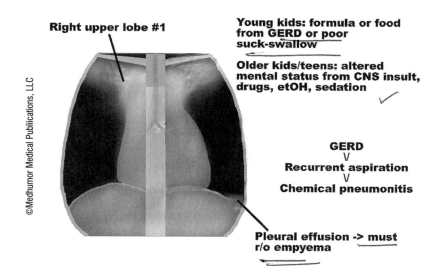

Right upper lobe #1

Young kids: formula or food from GERD or poor suck-swallow

Older kids/teens: altered mental status from CNS insult, drugs, etOH, sedation

GERD
V
Recurrent aspiration
V
Chemical pneumonitis

Pleural effusion -> must r/o empyema

©Medhumor Medical Publications, LLC

Younger Children

This is common in children with GERD or neurological conditions that include a poor gag reflex or suck swallow mechanism

Older Children

In older children aspiration pneumonia would be associated with altered mental status, for example drug overdose.

Look in the right upper lobe for aspiration pneumonia. If there is an associated pleural effusion consider a co-diagnosis of emphysema.

Bacterial Pneumonia

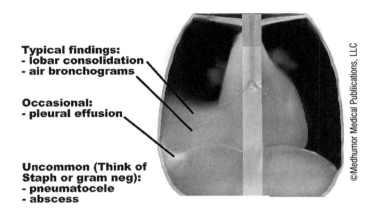

Typical findings:
- lobar consolidation
- air bronchograms

Occasional:
- pleural effusion

Uncommon (Think of Staph or gram neg):
- pneumatocele
- abscess

©Medhumor Medical Publications, LLC

The typical findings include lobar consolidation, air bronchograms and occasionally pleural effusion

With Staph or gram negative pneumonia look for pneumatocele and/or abscess

Atelectasis

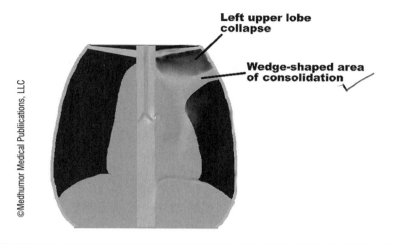

Left upper lobe collapse

Wedge-shaped area of consolidation

©Medhumor Medical Publications, LLC

Look for left upper lobe collapse and wedged shaped area of consolidation.

Di George's Syndrome

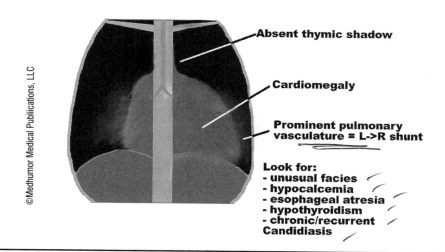

©Medhumor Medical Publications, LLC

Absent thymic shadow

Cardiomegaly

Prominent pulmonary
vasculature = L->R shunt

Look for:
- unusual facies
- hypocalcemia
- esophageal atresia
- hypothyroidism
- chronic/recurrent
Candidiasis

On Chest x-ray in Di George's Syndrome look for

1) Absent Thymic Shadow in an infant
2) Cardiomegaly
3) Prominent pulmonary Vasculare(which is due to L -‡ R shunting)

Additional findings would include a description of:

A) unusual facies
B) Hypocalcemia
C) Esophageal Atresia
D) Hypothyroidism
E) Candidiasis

Think of something

Hydrocarbon Pneumonia

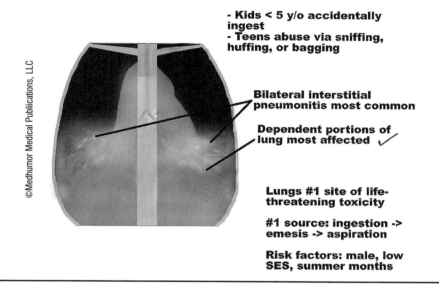

©Medhumor Medical Publications, LLC

- Kids < 5 y/o accidentally ingest
- Teens abuse via sniffing, huffing, or bagging

Bilateral interstitial pneumonitis most common

Dependent portions of lung most affected ✓

Lungs #1 site of life-threatening toxicity

#1 source: ingestion -> emesis -> aspiration

Risk factors: male, low SES, summer months

Typically will occur either with :

- Child younger than 5 after an accidental ingestion
- Teen sniffing glue

Clues in the history will include a child of lower socioeconomic status, during the summer, male.

You will typically be shown a CXR in a patient with the above history look for bilateral interstitial pneumonitis or diffuse infiltrates with the dependent portions most affected, i.e. the lung bases.

Necrotizing Enterocolitis

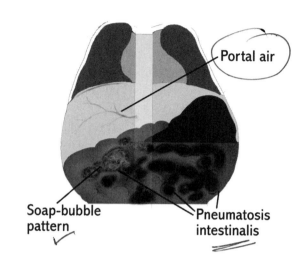

©Medhumor Medical Publiications, LLC

Portal air

Soap-bubble pattern

Pneumatosis intestinalis

Portal air, soap bubble pattern, pneumatosis intestinalis.

Typically seen in a premature newborn

PCP Pneumonia

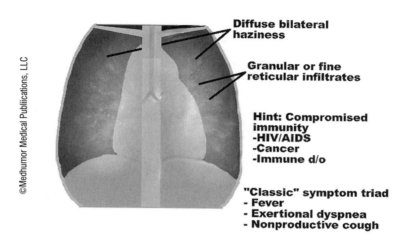

©Medhumor Medical Publications, LLC

Diffuse bilateral haziness

Granular or fine reticular infiltrates

Hint: Compromised immunity
-HIV/AIDS
-Cancer
-Immune d/o

"Classic" symptom triad
- Fever
- Exertional dyspnea
- Nonproductive cough

On CXR look for diffuse bilateral haziness, granular/fine reticular infiltrates,

The typical history will include a patient who is immunodeficient, typically a patient with AIDS or has another immuno disorder such as cancer

The classic triad for PCP pneumonia includes

    1) Fever

    2) Exertional Dyspnea

    3) Non-productive cough

Respiratory Distress Syndrome
aka Hyaline Membrane Disease

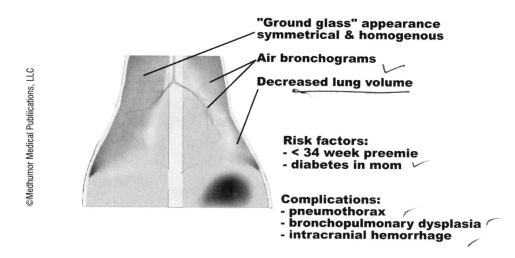

"Ground glass" appearance symmetrical & homogenous

Air bronchograms

Decreased lung volume

©Medhumor Medical Publications, LLC

Risk factors:
- < 34 week preemie
- diabetes in mom

Complications:
- pneumothorax
- bronchopulmonary dysplasia
- intracranial hemorrhage

DEFINITION

RDS is a result of *surfactant* deficiency at the alveolar level

RDS is also known as *hyaline membrane disease.*

LOOK FOR

Some of the typical adjectives to describe an infant with RDS would include grunting, tachypnea, nasal flaring, and chest retractions.

PERIL
WARNING

This is indistinguishable from the physical findings of the typical middle aged physician training for the triathlon, of getting up, getting the newspaper left in a neighbor's driveway and returning on time to change their infant' diaper without the aid of slippers.

PERIL
WARNING

RDS can be seen in full term infants therefore don't block it out as a possible diagnosis in a question involving a full term infant

---

The x-ray findings of RDS are virtually indistinguishable from Group B strep pneumonia. It will be the clinical features described that will allow you to differentiate the two.

The chest x-ray will show the classic ground glass appearance and air bronchograms.

Bronchiectasis

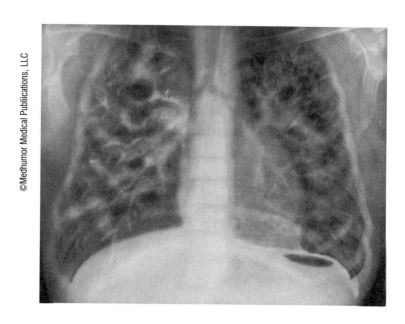

©Medhumor Medical Publications, LLC

 Bronchiectasis is due to dilation and destruction of large bronchi

Multiple cystic spaces (ring shadows), peribronchial fibrosis, and mild lung hyperexpansion (flattened hemidiaphragms)

Diffuse bronchiectasis, associated with cystic fibrosis, immune deficiencies, primary ciliary dyskinesia, and recurrent aspiration syndromes

Tension Pneumothorax

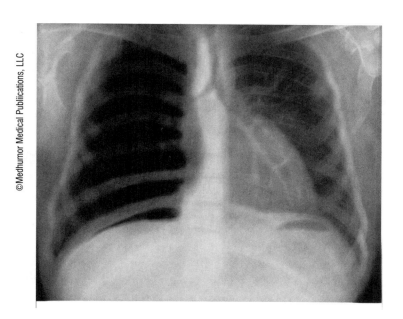

©Medhumor Medical Publications, LLC

The CXR findings depicted include

- Collapsed right lung: hyperlucent (black) with absent pulmonary markings
- Shift of mediastinum away from pneumothorax (to the left)
- Depression of ipsilateral (right) hemidiaphragm
- Well demarcated right and left main stem bronchi

Rheumatology

Subcutaneous Nodules

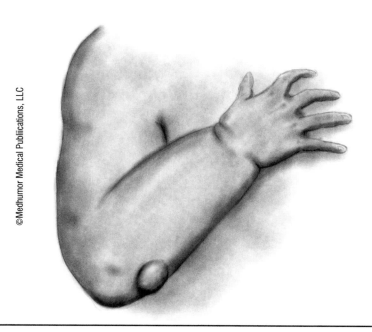

©Medhumor Medical Publications, LLC

 The drawing depicts

- A firm, nontender, mobile subcutaneous nodule
- Subcutaneous nodules are most often present at bony prominences, extensor surfaces, or adjacent to joints
- These are the most common extra-articular manifestations of rheumatoid arthritis.

Subcutaneous nodules are **not** pathognomonic of rheumatoid arthritis. They can also be seen in lupus, and even in healthy children.

Section 2:
Picture Perfect
Color

Dermatology

Acrodermatitis Enteropathica

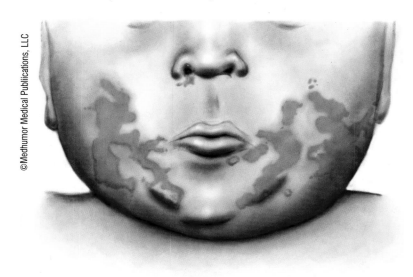

©Medhumor Medical Publications, LLC

The drawing illustrates the characteristic skin lesions include a periorificial and acral vesiculobullous eruption leading to scaly, sharply demarcated crusted plaques.

Acrodermatitis enteropathica is due to zinc deficiency. The deficiency can be due to nutritional deficiency or a congenital form is due to a defect in zinc absorption

Manifestations of the disease typically present when the affected infant is weaned from breast feeding.

Erythema Chronicum Migrans

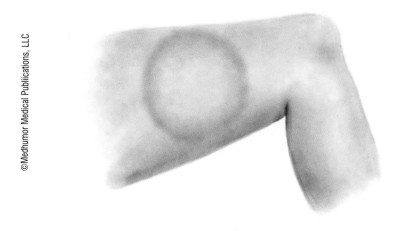

©Medhumor Medical Publications, LLC

MEDIAL THIGH

The illustration demonstrates the classic bullseye lesion of the erythema chronicum migrans. This is the rash associated with Lyme disease.

The rash typically begins as a red papule that expands peripherally and clears centrally

Erythema Marginatum

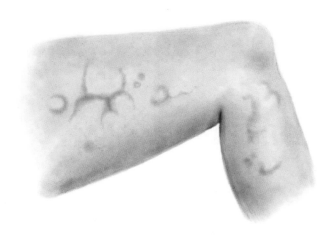

©Medhumor Medical Publications, LLC

MEDIAL THIGH

The illustration demonstrates the classic presentation of erythema marginatum which is associated with rheumatic fever.

Erythema marginatum is characterized by pink rings on the trunk and inner surfaces of the arms and legs which are evanescent for several months. The rings are barely raised and are non-pruritic.

Erythema Nodosum

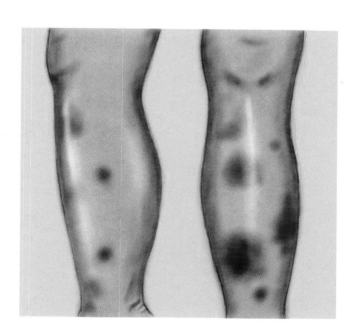

©Medhumor Medical Publications, LLC

The classic red-purplish painful, tender lumps typically presented on the extensor surfaces, i.e. the shins. They consist of subcutaneous nodules and are due to inflammation of the subcutaneous fat tissue.

It is associated with the use of oral contraceptives as well as inflammatory bowel disease. The most common precipitant is group A beta- hemolytic strep.

It can be mistaken for child abuse especially on the exam if there are red herring hints dropped luring you into making a diagnosis of child abuse.

Facial Angiofibromas

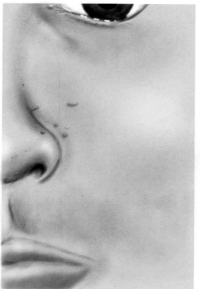

©Medhumor Medical Publiications, LLC

Facial angiofibromas as outlined in the illustration are seen in patients with tuberous sclerosus

These are not observed at birth. They appear between ages 3-5.

Lichen Sclerosus et Atrophicus

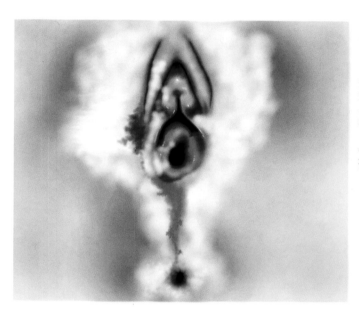

©Medhumor Medical Publiications, LLC

As depicted in the illustration , lichen sclerosus is characterized by atrophic depigmented tissue in the anogenital area. The atrophic tissue often has an hour glass appearance as depicted here.

It is often mistaken for sexual abuse. It is easy to be diverted into believing this on the exam. Watch for the specific findings of lichen sclerosus. If this is the diagnosis then the correct management would be reassurance since in most cases this is self limited resolving with the onset of menses.

Local Reaction to Immunotherapy

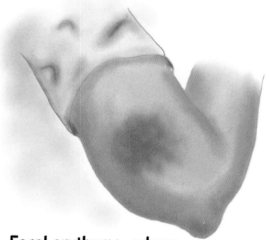

©Medhumor Medical Publications, LLC

- Focal erythema, edema
- Poor predictor of subsequent systemic reaction

The illustration demonstrates a local reaction to immunotherapy. Clearly in addition to the photograph you will need to also be presented with a clinical history suggesting the diagnosis.

Nevus Sebaceous
of Jadassohn

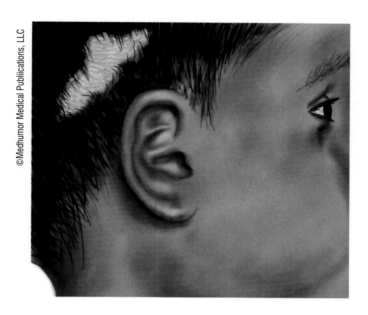

©Medhumor Medical Publications, LLC

DEFINITION

Nevus Sebaceous of Jadassohn is a hamartomatous disorder, which consists of immature sebaceous glands.

ANSWER REVEALED

As demonstrated in the illustration you should look for a hairless yellow- orange patch. It will be described as velvet like plaque.

INSIDER TIPS

These lesions have the potential to transform into a malignancy. This occurs a whopping 15% of the time after puberty.

Pityriasis Alba

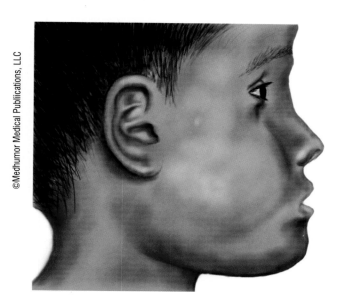

©Medhumor Medical Publications, LLC

Pityriasis Alba is a hypopigmented dermatitis typically involving the face. It is seen primarily in preadolescent children.

The illustration depicts a classic example of **pityriasis alba**. The patient is a preadolescent with facial hypopigmentation.

Pityriasis Alba is self limited with no known etiology. It is primarily seen on the face. Consider this if you are presented with a hypopigmented lesion on the face.

Tinea versicolor is caused by a yeast-like organism. Treatment is with antifungal creams and often recurs even after treatment. The lesions usually effect the upper chest, back, and shoulders.

Tinea versicolor can be hypopigmented or fawn colored. Lesions can coalesce.

Tinea Versicolor

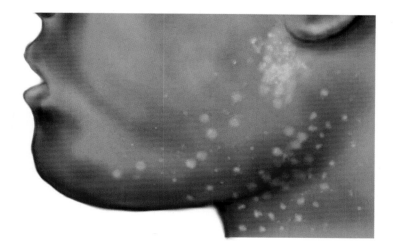

P. alba
AD — P. rosacea
↓
christmas
Tree
pattern

DEFINITION Tinea versicolor and Pityriasis versicolor are synonymous. It is hypopigmentation or fawn colored scaly macules. The macules are typically located on the back and can be confluent.

ANSWER REVEALED Although it frequently appears on the back, Tinea versicolor can occur on the face. In the illustration it is important to note that the lesions are not confluent.

INSIDER TIPS On Woods Lamp examination the lesions appear to be yellow fluorescent. Treatment is with topical antifungal cream. Recurrence rate after treatment is frequent.

EITHER OR CHOICES Pityriasis Alba, also consists of hypopigmented patches. However there is no known etiology and the conditions is self limited. In addition pityriasis Alba usually appears on the face, especially on the exam.

Stevens Johnson Syndrome

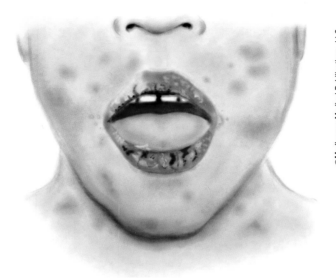

©Medhumor Medical Publiications, LLC

DEFINITION

Stevens Johnson syndrome is also known as **erythema multiforme major**. It is a hypersensitivity reaction to *infection, medications* or *illness*.

The rash begins as macules evolving into vesicles, papules, urticarial plaques, bullae or confluent erythema.

ANSWER REVEALED

The illustration demonstrates the oral mucosal involvement frequently seen in Stevens- Johnson syndrome. The lesions on the skin represent the target lesions. Erythematous macules are also seen in Stevens Johnson Syndrome.

Target lesions as well as mucous membrane involvement are the classic findings.

INSIDER TIPS

There are other important points you are expected to know to help you recognize Stevens Johnson Syndrome.

The bullous lesions can rupture resulting in denuded skin leading to infection.

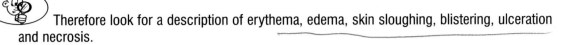 Therefore look for a description of erythema, edema, skin sloughing, blistering, ulceration and necrosis.

Consider Stevens Johnson Syndrome if they show you bullous lesions with a casual mention that the child recently was on an antibiotic such as amoxicillin.

Urticaria

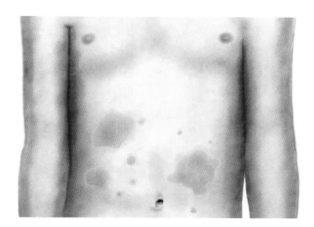

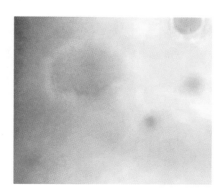

The illustration depicts edematous pink red lesions of varying size. This should be enough for you to identify the diagnosis as hives. They could present some additional history or ask you how you would manage the rash illustrated.

The treatment would consist of identifying the offending agent if possible and discontinuing exposure. Antihistamines and/or steroids would be among the possible treatment options.

Tinea Pedis
(Athlete's Foot)

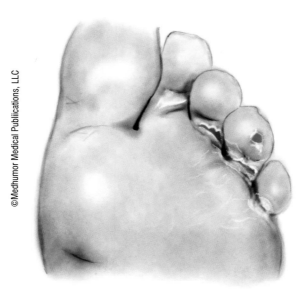

©Medhumor Medical Publications, LLC

 The key features depicted are pruritic scaly fissures including intertriginous tissue. The skin is often cracked and sometimes bleeding as in this illustration.

You will be expected to differentiate tinea pedis from **juvenile plantar dermatosis**.

Juvenile plantar dermatosis is essentially "wet soggy foot dermatitis ". Juvenile plantar dermatosis spares the interdigital tissue and this is the best way to differentiated it from tinea pedis.

Pitted Keratolysis

©Medhumor Medical Publications, LLC

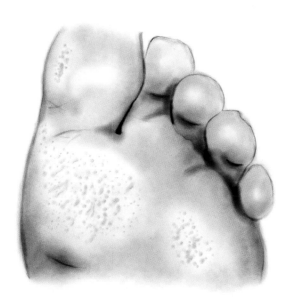

DEFINITION

Pitted keratolysis affects those who sweat profusely (hyperhidrosis). This is especially so if the patient were occlusive shoes such as the plastic tuxedo variety. It is caused by Corynebacteria, and/or the bacteria Dermatophilus congolensis.

INSIDER TIPS

Yes their feet smell so bad they could empty a room full of vultures attending a manure conference.

THE DIVERSION

As demonstrated in the illustration the sole of the foot appears white with clusters of punched-out pits. The appearance is more dramatic when the feet are wet.

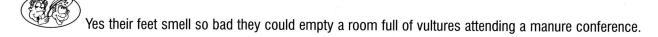

EITHER OR

Notice the different appearance between this and athlete's foot.

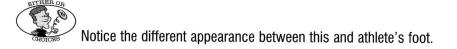

ENT

Goiter

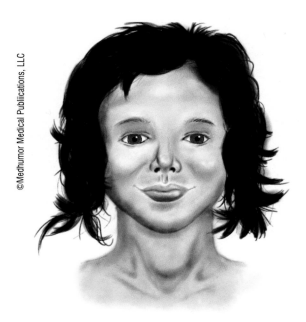

©Medhumor Medical Publications, LLC

The key features in the illustration include a diffuse, soft, symmetrical enlargement. This would be consistent with a thyroid goiter

They might throw in that the mass moves when the patient swallows. Additional physical findings might include a bruit on auscultation.

Mastoiditis

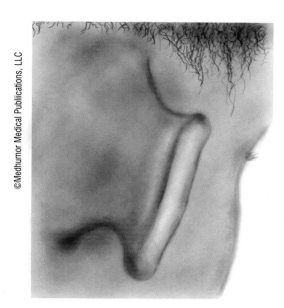

©Medhumor Medical Publications, LLC

The important features of mastoiditis in the illustration includes tenderness and erythema over the mastoid process along with displacement of the outer ear and pinna.

Parotiditis

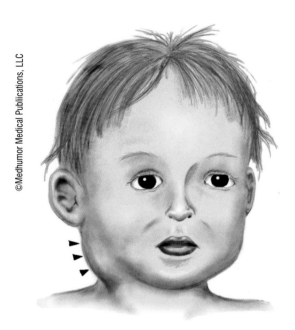

©Medhumor Medical Publications, LLC

 The important features to note in the drawing is pre-auricular swelling just under the angle of the mandible.

Parotid swelling can be due to several etiologies including:

∑• Mumps
∑• Parotid duct stone
∑• Staph infection

Genetics

Rubinstein-Taybi

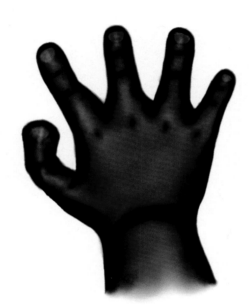

©Medhumor Medical Publications, LLC

Demonstrated here is the broad based thumb typical of Rubinstein - Taybi. They might also portray broad based great toe. If you see this in a picture picking the correct answer should be a slam dunk.

Achondroplasia Trident Hand

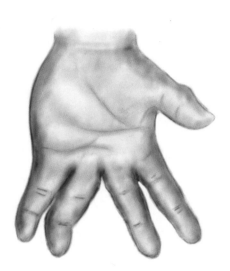

Heme, Onc

272

Kasabach-MerrittSyndrome

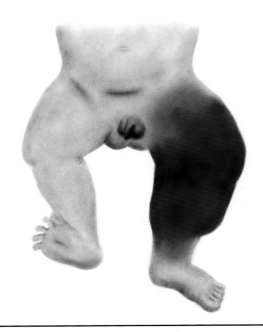

©Medhumor Medical Publications, LLC

 The illustration demonstrates the results the large tumor that consists of overgrown hemangioma. In this case the growth was rapid involving a large portion of the lower extremity.

This can result in thrombocytopenia and abnormal bleeding which can become life threatening.

---

1 In osteogenic sarcoma it can be a combination of lytic and sclerotic lesions however if pressed to make a choice lytic would be the correct choice.

Vitamin B12 Deficiency

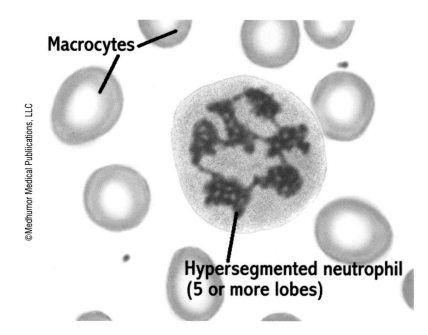

The blood smear depicts the typical findings seen in Vitamin B12 deficiency including macrocytes and hypersegmented neutrophils.

Neonatology

Congenital Candidiasis

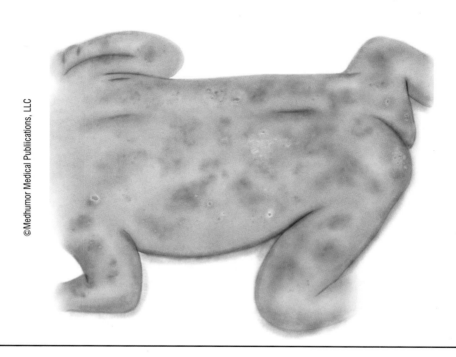

©Medhumor Medical Publications, LLC

Congenital candidiasis presents as a generalized scaly papulovesicular eruption.

Typicals the infection results from ascending maternal infection.

Congenital CMV

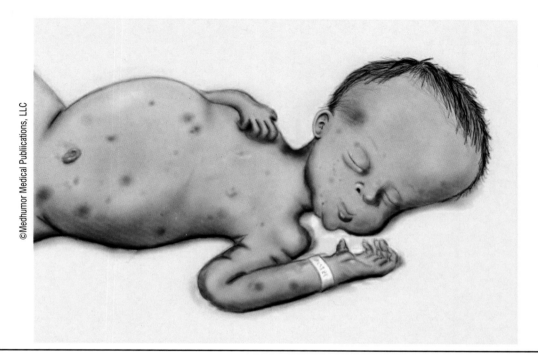

©Medhumor Medical Publications, LLC

Blueberry muffin baby

Diaper Dermatitis

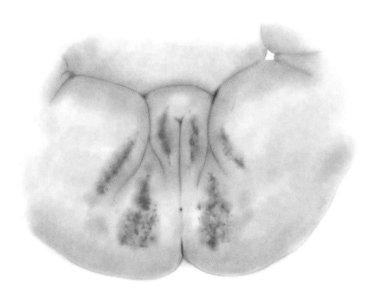

©Medhumor Medical Publications, LLC

 Some of the important features that will help you recognize diaper dermatitis:

- Chafing and erythema
- Primarily involvement is " convex" surfaces in the diaper area
- Creases are spared.

Seborrheic Dermatitis

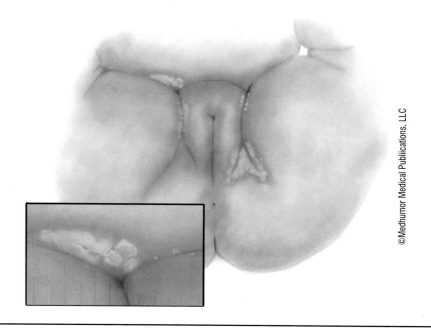

©Medhumor Medical Publications, LLC

The important characteristics noted in the illustration greasy scales and papules concentrated in the creases

Concentration in the creases is an important way to differentiating seborrheic dermatitis from diaper dermatitis.

Erythema Toxicum Neonatorum

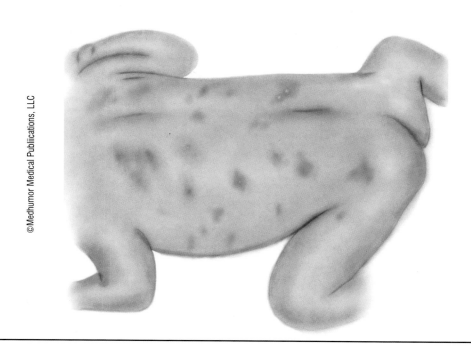

©Medhumor Medical Publications, LLC

Erythema toxicum neonatorum or "E tox" as it is commonly known is typically shown as whitish to yellowish-white vesicles surrounded by an erythematous base. The rash is typically generalized as demonstrated in the illustration.

Eosinophils

Neonatal Herpes

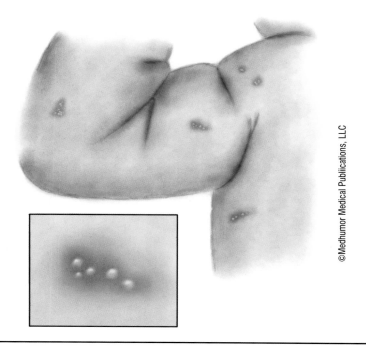

©Medhumor Medical Publiications, LLC

Neonatal herpes presents as grouped vesicles and/or pustules on the trunk as illustrated here. It can also be seen on the scalp and the extremities.

The lesions typically present between the third to sixth days of life.

It is typically acquired as an ascending infection during the birth process. Often it is a maternal primary infection with there being no previous history of genital herpes. In fact a previous history of genital herpes will never be part of the presenting history on the boards when presented with an infant with congenital herpes.

Transient Neonatal Pustular Melanosis

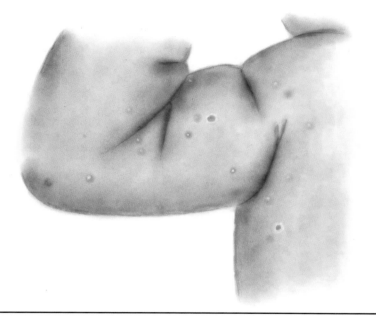

©Medhumor Medical Publications, LLC

 Transient neonatal pustular melanosis is a benign rash seen at birth. It is seen more often in African-American newborns than white newborns.

The typical presentation are vesiculopustules or ruptured pustules surrounded by scaly skin.

Although similar to erythema toxicum, you will not see an erythematous base in transient neonatal pustular melanosis.

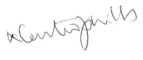

Ophthalmology

Aniridia

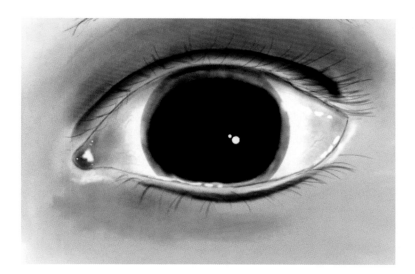

©Medhumor Medical Publications, LLC

 Aniridia is the incomplete formation of the iris. You will be presented with an eye where the iris is dilated.

 Aniridia is associated with Wilms tumor and Beckwith –Wiedemann syndrome.

WAGR

Chalazion

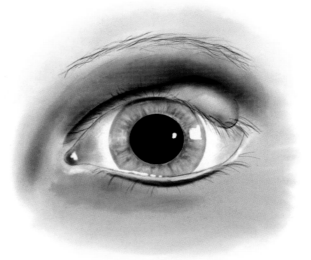

©Medhumor Medical Publications, LLC

A chalazion is a slowly enlarging lipogranuloma on the eyelid formed by inflammation of the glands. These nodules are often recurrent.

Initial treatment is warm compresses and sometime antibiotic eyedrops.

It will typically be described as a slowly growing non-tender mass.

Usually there is no erythema or tenderness.

Hordeolum

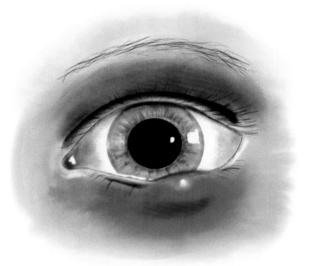

©Medhumor Medical Publications, LLC

A hordeolum usually represents an infection and is red and inflamed.

A **hordeolum** is red, tender and typically infected. Staph aureus is usually the infectious agent.

A **chalazion** is typically non –erythematous, non tender, and not infected.

Chorioretinitis

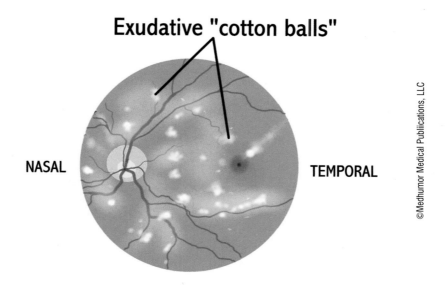

Exudative "cotton balls"

NASAL

TEMPORAL

©Medhumor Medical Publications, LLC

The most common cause of infection induced chorioretinitis is congenital toxoplasmosis.

The second most common cause of infection induced chorioretinitis is congenital CMV virus.

Coloboma

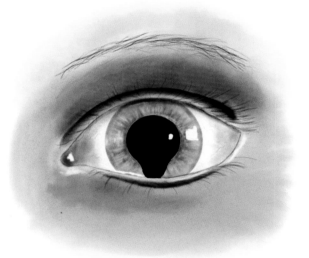

©Medhumor Medical Publications, LLC

 A coloboma is a cleft or split in the iris. This is what is depicted in the drawing.

Although coloboma can be associated with CHARGE syndrome most cases are not associated with other abnormalities.

Leukocoria

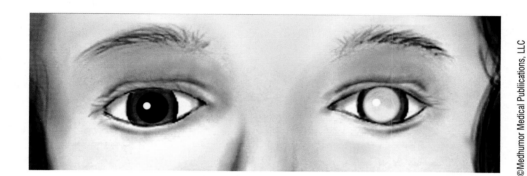

©Medhumor Medical Publilcations, LLC

Leukocoria is a white pupillary reflex. Simply it means something within the eye is blocking light from reflecting off the retina.

While there can be many causes the two to keep in mind are congenital cataracts and retinoblastoma depending on the historical context you are presented with.

Lisch Nodules

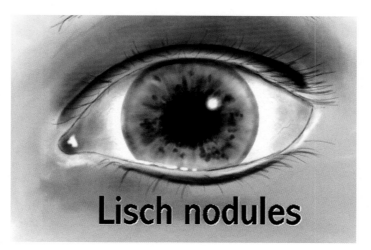

Lisch nodules

©Medhumor Medical Publiications, LLC

Lisch nodules are tan or benign tumors of the iris less than 2 mm in diameter. It is associated with neurofibromatosis type 1.

Retinal Detachment

Few vessels

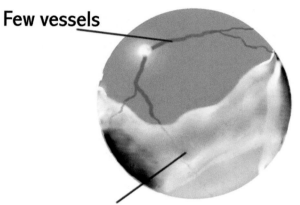

©Medhumor Medical Publications, LLC

Retinal tear, flap, or corrugated folds

ANSWER REVEALED

The drawing depicting retinal detachment includes a paucity of vessels. Watch for the retinal flap. The view looks like the eye is partitioned into 2 parts.

LOOK FOR

Watch for a history of trauma and/or participation in contact sports.

If you see a funduscopic exam that looks like an aerial view of Mars obscured by clouds you are probably looking at retinal detachment.

Retinal Hemorrhage

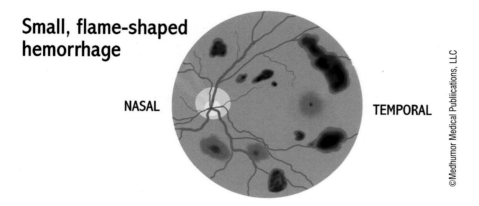

**Small, flame-shaped
hemorrhage**

NASAL   TEMPORAL

©Medhumor Medical Publications, LLC

The drawing demonstrates the classic picture of retinal hemorrhage on funduscopic exam including flame shaped hemorrhages.

Watch for a history or suspicion of child abuse. This a pathognomic sign of " shaken baby syndrome"

Retinitis Pigmentosa

Optic disc w/ "waxy pallor"

NASAL

TEMPORAL

©Medhumor Medical Publications, LLC

Narrow arterioles

Retinal pigment
deposition

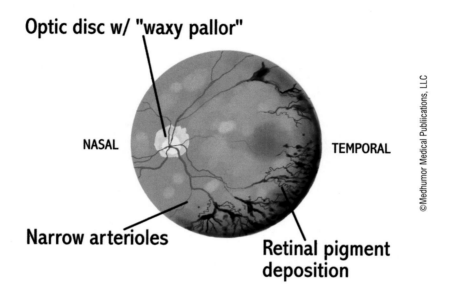

ANSWER REVEALED   The illustration depicts the funduscopic findings which correlate with the retinal degeneration of retinitis pigmentosa.

LOOK FOR   Initially starts out with peripheral vision loss, then night blindness and ultimately central visual deficits. It is also an inherited condition and therefore tends to run in families. Therefore watch for a family history of visual deficits and blindness.

Retinopathy of Prematurity

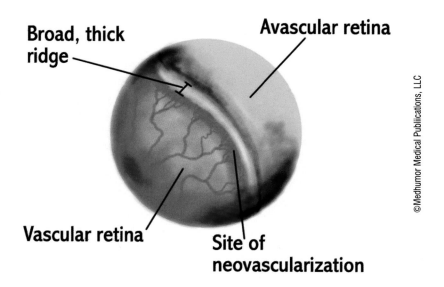

Broad, thick ridge

Avascular retina

Vascular retina

Site of neovascularization

©Medhumor Medical Publications, LLC

In recognizing retinopathy of prematurity watch for the retina being partly avascular with a ridge separating it from the vascular component. Near the ridge will be evidence of neovascularization.

Orthopaedics

Osgood-Schlatter Disease

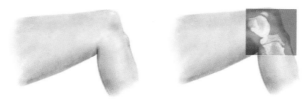

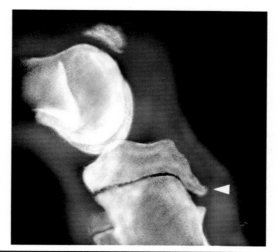

Osgood –Schlatter is due to inflammation over the anterior tubercle at the point of insertion of the patellar tendon.

It presents as intermittent pain after weight bearing activities

The x-ray findings coupled with the appropriate history is diagnostic for this condition

Rheumatology

Dermatomyositis
(Heliotrope Rash)

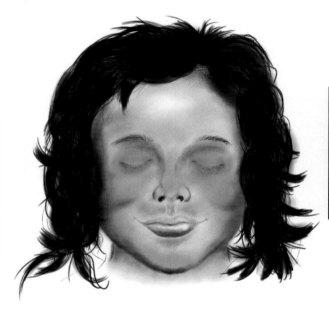 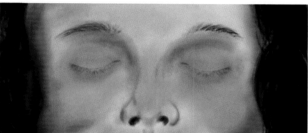

The typical heliotrope rash seen in dermatomyositis is a reddish purple facial rash manifesting primarily in the periorbital tissue. Edema is another component.

Additional findings not demonstrated in the illustrations includes *Gottron papules*, which are atrophic papules over the knuckles and sometimes the interphalangeal joints, knees and elbows.

The facial rash of dermatomyositis is similar to buttefly rash seen in lupus.

One important way to differentiated them is to look at the eyes.

In dermatomyositis, telangiectasia causes the " heliotrope "appearance of the eyelids.

In lupus the rash may involve the eyebrows, however the malar/butterfly rash will not involve the orbits.

SLE

(Malar or Butterfly Rash)

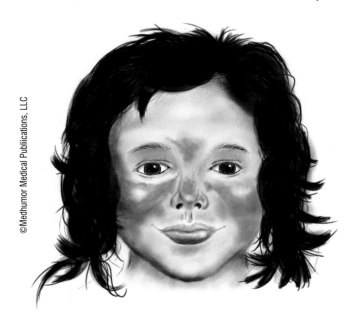

©Medhumor Medical Publications, LLC

 Note the following characteristics of the malar rash seen in SLE. It is a classic butterfly distribution. The rash is primarily erythematous papules.

The nasolabial and periorbital areas are spared.

Henoch Schoenlein Purpura

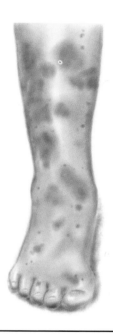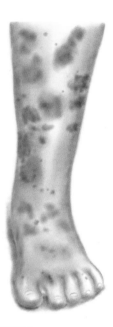

©Medhumor Medical Publications, LLC

The illustration demonstrates the palpable purpura associated with Henoch Schönlein purpura (HSP). The purpura are typically seen in "dependent "parts of the body. The typical location of the purpura in HSP is the lower extremities.

It is very easy to confuse these lesions with child abuse and on the exam they may drop diversionary hints leading you incorrectly concluding that child abuse is the correct diagnosis.

Kawasaki

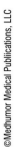

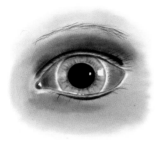

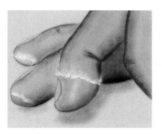

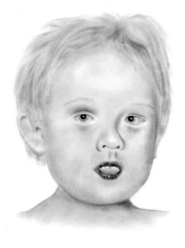

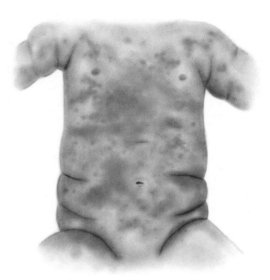

You could be shown any one of the following manifestations of Kawasaki disease or mucocutaneous lymph node syndrome.

Trunk – erythematous papular eruption

Lips – The cracked lips illustrated one of the mucous membrane manifestations of Kawasaki disease. Other mucous membrane manifestations would include strawberry tongue and erythema of the buccal mucosa.

Finger Tips – Desquamation of the fingertips is another classic manifestation of Kawasaki disease.

Non exudative conjunctivitis – is another important manifestation of Kawasaki disease. The key is to remember the conjunctivitis is non-exudative.

GU

Epididymo-Orchitis

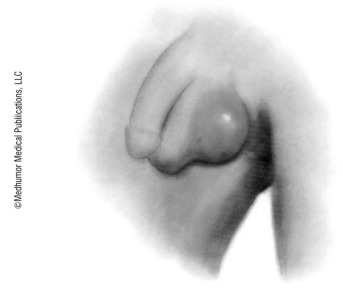

©Medhumor Medical Publications, LLC

Orchitis is an inflammatory process of the testes and epididymis.

It is important to distinguish between epididymitis and torsion of the testicle.

This distinction is usually made on clinical history or physical exam (description on the boards).

Inguinal Hernia

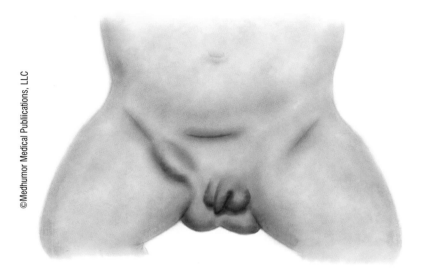

©Medhumor Medical Publications, LLC

If you are shown an infant with an inguinal mass as in the illustration the most likely diagnosis is an inguinal hernia.

Varicocele

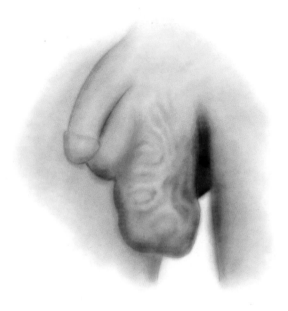

©Medhumor Medical Publications, LLC

A varicocele is a group of dilated veins. Pain is rarely a part of the presentation.

It looks very much like a bag of worms as depicted in the illustration.

Infectious Disease

Brown Recluse Spider Bite
(dermonecrotic arachnidism)

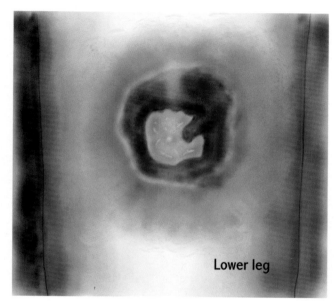
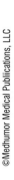

©Medhumor Medical Publications, LLC

Lower leg

The key features to watch out for as follows:

- Red, white and blue.
    - White center
    - Blue / purple surrounding the center
    - Red / erythematous rim

Extensive necrosis may result as well.

It can initially present as a painless lesion.

Bullous Impetigo

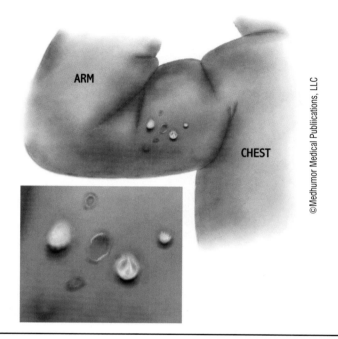

The illustration depicts the characteristic vesicles and pustules that develop into thin-walled bullae which rupture easily.

The lesions can then be covered by a yellow crust.

The face, trunk can be involved, and as illustrated here the extremities of infants and children are mainly affected.

Non Bullous Impetigo

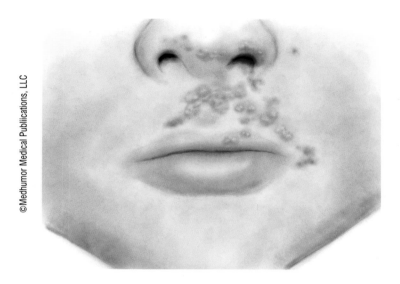

©Medhumor Medical Publications, LLC

 The illustration portrays the typical crusted honeycomb appearing lesions of non-bullous impetigo. Frequently it appears near the nose.

- Beta-hemolytic streptococcus usually produces **nonbullous impetigo**.
- Coagulase-positive staphylococcus aureus usually causes **bullous impetigo**.

Erythema Infectiosum

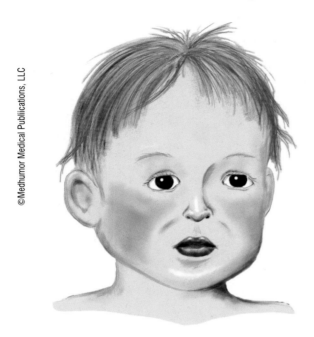

©Medhumor Medical Publications, LLC

Note the typical slapped cheek associated with erythema infectiosum also known as fifth disease. The rash typically appears after the fever has subsided.

Insider Tips

The nasolabial folds and circumoral area are spared.

Hand Foot Mouth
Coxsackie

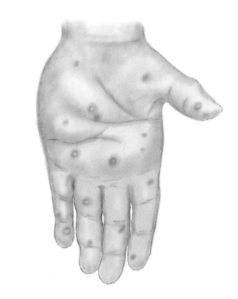

©Medhumor Medical Publications, LLC

The hand lesions in the illustration are typical for coxsackie, hand , foot, mouth disease. The lesions are oval gray-roofed vesicles against an erythematous base.

They could present you with additional information including a history of fever and mild lethargy.

The lesions do not have to appear on the hands, feet and mouth to make the diagnosis.

Herpes Zoster

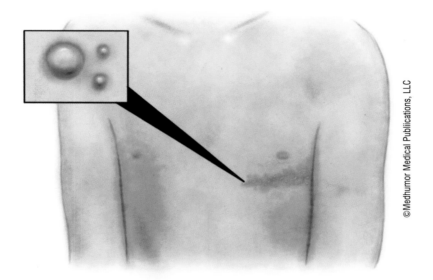

Herpes zoster manifests when the virus laying dormant in a sensory ganglion is reactivated. This results in a localized recurrence along a defined dermatome.

As demonstrated in the illustration, the key points to remember is that herpes zoster presents as grouped vesicles in a dermatome distribution. The distribution will be unilateral.

Of course herpes zoster is also known as shingles.

Infectious Mononucleosis Ampicillin Rash Mono

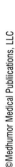
©Medhumor Medical Publications, LLC

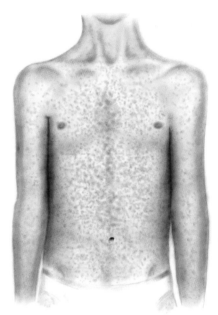

The illustration demonstrates a generalized erythematous papular rash seen in patients with infectious mono who are also taking penicillin or amoxicillin.

In addition to the photo they will have to present you with a history that hints at an underlying diagnosis of infectious mono in a patient on amoxicillin or penicillin.

Maculae Cerulea

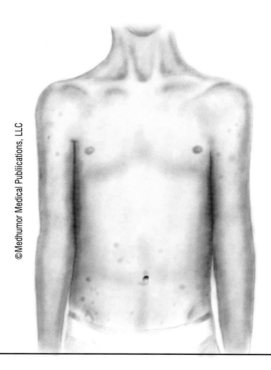

©Medhumor Medical Publications, LLC

Maculae cerulea is Latin for blue spots are a result or lice infestations.

The itching that accompanies lice infestation is an allergic reaction to a toxin in the saliva of the lice. Repeated bites can lead to a generalized skin eruption or inflammation which is depicted in the illustration.

Measles

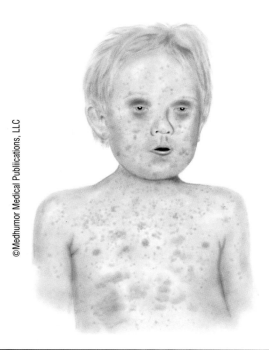

©Medhumor Medical Publiications, LLC

 The important characteristics of measles noted in this illustration include:

- Discrete maculopapular rash on the extremities
- Confluence of the rash on the trunk
- Morbilliform rash seen on day 3
- Conjunctivitis

 Not demonstrated here are the Koplik spots which are pathognomonic for measles. These are white dots seen on the erythematous buccal mucosa.

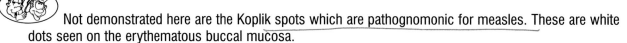 While Koplik spots are pathognomonic for measles its absence does not rule out measles.

Remember the 3 C's of measles

1) Cough
2) Coryza
3) Conjunctivitis

While Kawasaki disease can also present with a generalized rash and conjunctivitis, in measles the other salient features of Kawasaki disease will be absent. These features, specific for Kawasaki disease include fissured lips and peeling of the fingers.

Puncture Wound

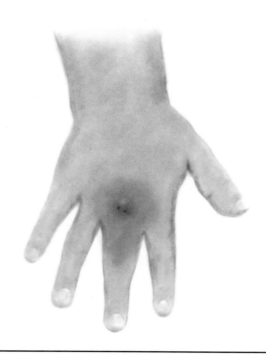

©Medhumor Medical Publications, LLC

 Note the portal of entry and the erythema consistent with rapidly spreading cellulitis.

Rocky Mountain Spotted Fever

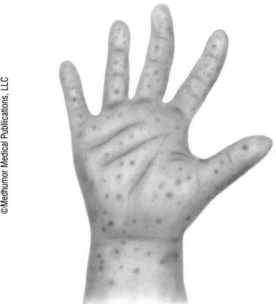

©Medhumor Medical Publications, LLC

The illustrations would be consistent with the physical findings of early rocky mountain spotted fever. The rash is an erythematous papulrar rash on the palms.

It can also start on the soles of the feet and the wrists

The rash typically spreads to the trunk within hours.

Rocky mountain spotted fever can present without the typical rash. However this is unlikely to occur on the boards.

Roseola

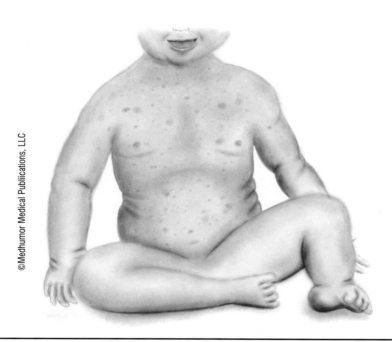

©Medhumor Medical Publications, LLC

The official name is roseola infantum and is typically caused by herpesvirus-6.

The illustration demonstrates the diffuse erythematous papular eruption diagnostic of roseola.

For those who are actually interested in such trivialities roseola is also known as sixth disease. The reason for this has something to do with the order in which the typical childhood viral illnesses were discovered and way too boring to get into now.

The rash appears on day 3-4 after the fever stops.

Scabies

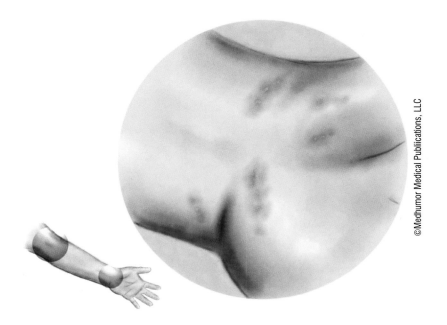

©Medhumor Medical Publications, LLC

Although tracking is not always present, it will likely be evident on any graphic depicted on the boards. It is *not* always present in interdigital tissue, especially in children.

The lesions may also appear to be excoriated and eczematous especially after chronic scratching.

Scarlet Fever

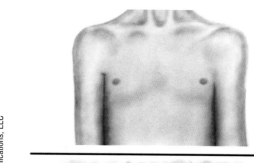
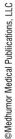
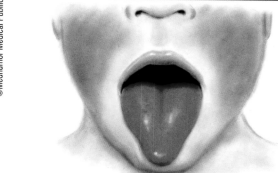

©Medhumor Medical Publications, LLC

The illustrations feature the strawberry tongue seen in scarlet fever as well as the classic sandpaper rash. The sandpaper rash might be described as a punctiform erythematous papular rash.

Additional findings not featured here would include Pastia sign which is red streaks on the skin folds

Smallpox vs Chickenpox

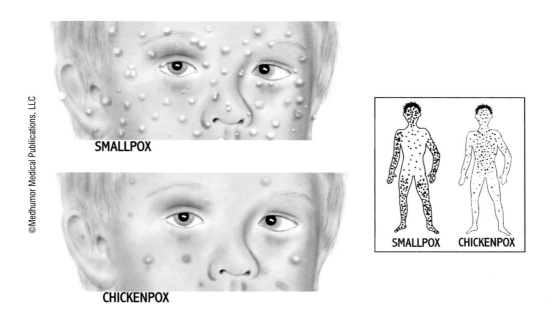

In the post 911 world you are expected to recognize manifestations of bioterrorism including smallpox.

Specifically you are expected to differentiate Variola (smallpox) from varicella (chickenpox)

 The illustration helps focus on how to differentiate them.

Regarding **distribution**:

Chickenpox – the rash is sparse distally and concentrated centrally. The face is typically spared.

Smallpox – the rash is sparse centrally and concentrated distally and on the face.

Chickenpox lesions are much more superficial than smallpox lesions.

Regarding **stage of development of individual lesions:**

ChickenPox – The lesions are in varying stages of development. Some lesions are scabbed over, some are vesicles, and some are pustules. This is even the case in the same region of the body.

Smallpox – all of the lesions are in the same stage of development, especially in the same area of the body.

In chickenpox lesions progress from macules to papules within 24 hours

In smallpox lesions progress from macules to papules over the course of days.

When is the patient contagious?

Chickenpox- A patient can be contagious prior to the appearance of the rash.

Smallpox- Patients with smallpox are only contagious when the signs and symptoms appear.

Staphylococcal Folliculitis

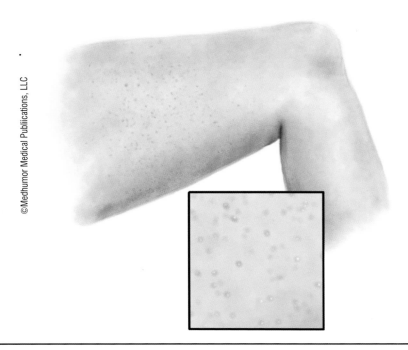

©Medhumor Medical Publications, LLC

 The important features to recognize are scattered small pustules involving areas where hair follicles are prominent.

Watch for a history of recent swimming in a public pool or hot tub.

Toxic Shock Syndrome

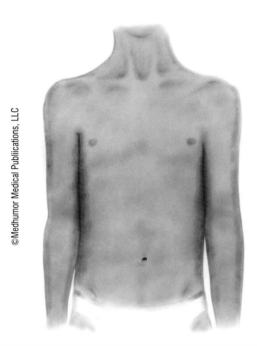

©Medhumor Medical Publications, LLC

Toxic shock syndrome is caused by a toxin producing strain of Staph aureus. It is potentially life threatening and the patient they present you with could be in the ICU.

The illustration demonstrates the diffuse macular/ scarlatiniform skin eruption seen in toxic shock syndrome.

They will likely need to present you with other findings to point to this diagnosis. This might include hypotension or something subtle like noting that the patient is female and her sexual maturity rating is 5. This would tip you off that she might be using tampons and is therefore at risk for toxic shock syndrome.

We Want Your Contributions

In an effort to keep **Pictures Worth a 100 Points**™ current, we will be publishing revised editions on a regular basis. We invite you to contribute your own:

- Topics you encountered on the exam that were troublesome and tricky to navigate
- Memory Aids
- Suggestions for topics
- New or little known facts

For each suggestion we use, we will send you a gift certificate towards our products and we will include your name in the acknowledgment section of our next edition.

We also welcome general comments on how helpful specific sections, including memory aids, were to you. Please let us know if you feel there are topics that could be left out or added to the book.

You can send your comments and contributions to us via e-mail to revisions@passtheboards.com or via mail to:

MedHumor Medical Publications
Attention: Pictures Worth a 100 Points Revisions
1127 High Ridge Rd., Suite 332
Stamford, CT. 06905

Faxes are also accepted at 203-323-9036.

Don't forget to visit our active web site at www.passtheboards.com for updated information, corrections, discussion groups, and other interactive mediums.